PSYCHOLOGICAL DISTRESS IN AGING

A Family Management Model

Donna R. Eyde, Ph.D.
Jay A. Rich, M.D.

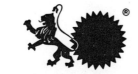

AN ASPEN PUBLICATION®
Aspen Systems Corporation
Rockville, Maryland
London
1983

Library of Congress Cataloging in Publication Data

Eyde, Donna R.
Psychological distress in aging.

Includes bibliographies and index.
1. Aged—Mental health services. 2. Aged—Home care.
I. Rich, Jay A. II. Title. [DNLM: 1. Mental disorders
—In old age. 2. Family therapy. 3. Mental health
services—In old age. 4. Mental disorders—Therapy.
WT 150 E97p]
RC451.4.A5E83 1983   362.8′2   82-16440
ISBN: 0-89443-667-8

Publisher: John Marozsan
Editorial Director: R. Curtis Whitesel
Managing Editor: Margot Raphael
Editorial Services: Scott Ballotin
Printing and Manufacturing: Debbie Collins

Library of Congress Catalog Card Number: 82-16440
ISBN: 0-89443-667-8

Printed in the United States of America

1 2 3 4 5

*This book is dedicated
to our grandparents, older
friends, and patients.*

Table of Contents

Acknowledgments

The seemingly individualistic task of writing a book serves merely to illuminate the interdependencies of ideas, authors, friends, and families. Two individuals deserve special commendation in this joint effort: Nancy Sullivan and Ted Winschief. Truly, without their technical support this text would not have been produced. A similar debt of gratitude is owed to our friends and families for their patience. Many individuals including our patients and their families contributed to the ideas within this text. In particular, Frank J. Menolascino, M.D., and Evelyn Runyon are teachers whom we would like to thank formally. Dr. Menolascino constantly admonished us to ''tell it the way it is,'' and Mrs. Runyon helped us understand the way it really is.

Introduction

The elderly in our society have been described as a disposable generation—inflexible, nonproductive, and burdensome. Families have been accused of doing the disposing by abandoning the old to the institutionalized care of nursing homes and high-rises. While widespread abandonment is a myth, the struggles of caregiving to older members are real. Families care but are unsure of how best to meet the needs of aging parents, aunts, or uncles while simultaneously satisfying a myriad of demands of carpools, jobs, spouses, and growing children. Families lack guidelines for appropriate caregiving, and older members lack role clarity for seeking and receiving care. All generations lack critical information to meet the developmental challenges of later adulthood. The transitions inherent in the human life span hold the promise for growth as well as the potential for loss and pathology. Families must be helped to separate the good from the bad, the normal from the nonnormal, and the atypical from the predictable.

Family systems are characterized by change and readjustment as individual members negotiate the various life stages. An individual adolescent matures, develops beginning life interests, and leaves home. Young adults become newlyweds, parents, and active community members directing their energies to the larger society. Concurrently, their parents are engaged in their own psychosocial development as they accept the new roles of grandparents, in-laws, wise community leaders, and mentors. Older family members retire or begin second careers, necessitating more readjustment of the relative position and roles of other family members. The family system ripples with developmental changes and in most cases continues to readjust in a healthy fashion.

Failure to incorporate and perhaps even to value individual change among members leads to derailment of the family life cycle and stagnation of individual development. Failure to accept and support adolescent development increases the chances of a family maintaining a rebellious immature young adult member. Failure to accept the early life role of parenting after the birth of children derails the cycle of nurture and support for dependent children. Failure to accept the midlife roles of increasing responsibility and vocation/career achievement delays individual development and strains the family ability to compensate. Likewise, failure to adjust to the aging process of later adulthood impedes the evolution of the entire family life cycle.

The quality, degree, and type of attachment between individual family members change as each member negotiates individual life changes and the family life cycle readjusts. Family relationships provide the necessary milieu and momentum for continuous growth throughout the life span. Clearly, the total dependence of the infant necessitates a supportive family milieu. The dependencies, expectations, and needs of other ages such as childhood, adolescence, and early adult life also reflect on a supportive family milieu. Middle and late adult life results in a differing constellation of dependencies as well as aspirations and expectations. The developmental changes and demands of these later stages may differ but the need for a supportive family milieu continues despite our culture's failure to recognize or popularize this need.

Much of the psychological distress associated with the aging process and the evident unmet mental health needs of older persons is associated with adaptive failures in the transitional tasks of later life and with a lack of the necessary milieu to aid adjustment. Aging is a normal growth process, and old age is a normal stage in human development. Yet, mounting evidence suggests that the incidence of psychopathology increases steadily with each decade of life. Organic brain diseases become more prevalent after age 60, and individuals over 65 are the group most susceptible to mental illness. When the present trends of mental health needs among the aged are compared to the available professional care providers, it is evident that the majority of elderly people who need assistance will never be served by professionals unless methods of delivering mental health services are drastically altered. However, all will live, change, and die within a family system.

Only a small percentage of Americans over 65 live in alternative care facilities or without a family. The great majority of older persons depend upon their family to provide them with a sense of belonging and a sense of connectedness to the larger society. The family remains a key resource even for nonimpaired older persons who are successfully adapting to changes in physical health, social roles, relationships, cognitive functioning, and emotional demands. Older persons vary in their relative adjustment to changes; families vary greatly in natural resources, available coping strategies, and degree of commitment for caregiving. Some authors observe that certain family personalities may in fact deter or impede satisfactory adjustment to old age while others facilitate transitions.

Families face conflicting developmental demands and must balance their own needs against the responsibility of responding appropriately to the needs of aging members. This balancing act sometimes must be performed for one or more sets of parents or grandparents at the same moment when adult children are confronting their own developmental changes. The balance between affiliation needs, dependencies, and independence is often precarious.

A minor stress such as illness or accident, which may be a symptom of a developmental stressor (Hadley, Jacob, Milliones, Caplain, & Spitz, 1974), tips the scale, precipitating additional symptoms in other family members and leading to premature placement of the older impaired member.

Dependency is a common and pervasive influence as well as a cohesive social force in family systems (Goldfarb, 1974). However, if adult children fail to accept filial maturity (Neugarten, 1976) and to recognize that aging parents need to depend upon them, without forfeiting all personal decision-making freedom, then both generations are left feeling uncertain, angry, and frustrated. Members of the family system are confused about how best to help themselves and the older person.

The issue becomes more serious when one considers that shrinking public service resources and an expanding aged population will require increased participation by families at a time when most families are unsure of what to do. The number of generations within a family system are increasing due to longevity, marriage, and child-bearing patterns; however, the shrinking birthrate is reducing the number of kin in an absolute sense.

It is obvious that since the shortage of personnel prohibits direct service to all aged in need, the helping professions must assume greater responsibility for providing relevant information to be used in placement decisions and more indirect family-centered treatment. The family should know which needs could or should be met within a family. How these needs may be met, when and where outside helping services should be solicited are pressing concerns for today's middle generation; the answers will shape the contours of caregiving patterns for future generations.

This book is offered to help meet the challenges of growing older in America, by providing professional reference materials on family-centered treatment of the psychological stresses of aging. Specific procedures for practitioners helping families respond to the complexities of needs are described and evaluated. The focus of this book is on the family as a treatment milieu in meeting many secondary mental health needs of older persons and on the family as a case manager of the treatment resources needed to meet special, less predictable needs of impaired older individuals.

Naturalistic research suggests that the habilitative potential of the family milieu is circumscribed by several important constructs: (1) a life-span model of mental health needs and later adult development; (2) a functional analysis of biological, psychological, and sociological variables associated with a given mental health problem; and (3) a continuum and continuity of care options. It is necessary to consider simultaneously the evolution of the family system itself and the stages of development attained by the individual members who complement the family system. This view must be further refined by attention to biopsychosocial variables operating individually and collectively within the family relational patterns. Mental health in many senses is indicative of balance or equilibrium between the system's adaptive demands and the adaptive capacity of the members responding within the system. Interventions must be both holistic and individually prescriptive. The authors remain optimistic concerning the power of the family to respond to the needs of its members, preserve its own necessary boundaries, and integrate both past and future generations. Steady unremitting decline in individuals and disruptions of family systems are neither inevitable nor natural outcomes of the aging process.

The authors have attempted to provide health care and related professionals with a systematic approach to the identification, management, and treatment of psychological stresses and psychopathologies of older persons within a family system. Since it is important to maximize the mental health of any person at any point from birth to death, practical techniques are offered to bridge some of the gaps between theory and experience in prevention of psychological distress as well as in maintaining mental wellness. The escalating mental health problems among the aged create an urgency to translate theoretical positions and empirical findings into programmatic solutions. Consequently, it is our sincere wish that the guidelines offered throughout this text are subjected to scrutiny, filtered through the net of individual experience, and applied in the most meaningful fashion by the front-line worker.

REFERENCES

Goldfarb, A.V. Minor maladjustment in the aged. In S. Arieti & E.B. Brody (Eds.), *American handbook of psychiatry* (Vol. 3). New York: Basic Books, 1974.

Haldey, T.R., Jacob, T., Milliones, J., Caplain, J., & Spitz, D. The relationship between family developmental crisis and the appearance of symptoms in a family member. *Family Process,* 1974, *13,* 207–214.

Neugarten, B. Adaptation and the life cycle. *The Counseling Psychologist,* 1976, *6,* 16–20.

Chapter 1

Surviving in America

CURRENT CHALLENGES FOR FAMILIES WITH OLDER MEMBERS

Several factors actively contribute to the current and future demands on families with aging members. There are more older people proportionally as well as numerically. The old are considerably older than ever before in history. More people are confronting the developmental tasks of later life in a highly complex and rapidly changing sociopolitical climate. Mental health needs are increasing against a backdrop of shortages in trained personnel as well as personal and public resources. There are real and theoretical conflicts over retirement ages and a lack of clarity in roles and responsibilities. Families and their personal mental health needs are as varied as the conditions of their dependent members. The aging of our population is bringing new distresses for family systems. The normlessness of old age is becoming more evident at a time when our very notion of family is changing. Families are being structured in unfamiliar ways. Four- and five-generation families are more common along with increased divorce and remarriage rates. Reconstituted families, blended families, and "families of choice" are more visible in the social order along with a proliferation of specialized therapies to help variant forms succeed.

Surviving in America may increasingly depend upon professional responsiveness to emergent demands for innovative, cost-effective, specialized family-centered mental health services, especially for older members at a time when professionalism is overextended and a bit suspect. The family is the first and most critical link in a continuum of mental health services. Families are the informal case managers, record keepers, and information repositories, providing continuity of care for impaired members. The family system is the primary articulator of mental health needs across the life span of individual family members and should participate more actively in the decision-making process if families and we are to meet successfully the challenges of caring for an aging nation.

Mental Health Needs and the Life Span

The United States has become an aged nation for the first time in history, with more than 11.7 percent of its population over the age of 65. By the turn of the century, approximately 12 percent, or about 32 million individuals, will be over age 65 (Redick & Taube, 1980). Each day, the population of individuals over age 65 swells by approximately 1,600 persons. Biomedical and psychosocial problems associated with the aging process affect or will affect every family in the nation. Recent testimony before the special congressional committee on aging revealed that the elderly appear to be disproportionately subject to psychological distress. People in later life have the highest suicide rate and prevalence of mental disorders, consume more drugs, and exhibit more insidious and complex alcohol abuse than any other age group in the country (Klerman, 1980). Moreover, if present trends continue, about 80 percent of the elderly who need assistance for emotional and mental problems will never be served (Butler, 1978).

The gradual decline of physical abilities even in healthy elderly, interacts with psychological and sociological changes to make late-life adjustments extremely difficult, creating a larger at-risk population. The medical, personal, and social needs of the healthy and impaired aged are truly diverse. Meaningful responses to these needs must be equally diverse, flexible, and collaborative. Human growth and development is itself a diverse and dynamic process. The individual life cycle is marked by a changing self with changing needs. There are evident similarities in the ways in which individuals negotiate the developmental task along the life cycle; there are also significant differences. The groups of healthy and impaired aged reflect the similarities as well as the differences in human growth processes.

While there is no satisfactory theory of personality growth across a life span, Erikson (1959) was among the first to view the mental health needs of an individual in terms of a life cycle of developmental stages. The developmentalist approach was soon applied to a number of human problem areas, e.g., cognitive growth (Piaget, 1954, 1963, 1972), moral growth (Kohlberg, 1964, 1969, 1973), social attachment (Kalish & Knudtson, 1976), and psychosocial growth (Schaie, 1977-78). The developmentalist position maintains that each individual changes in complex ways throughout the life span. These changes are reflected in stages of development that are successive and sequentially organized. Each age or stage has general qualities that most individuals achieve at an approximate chronological age. Failure to integrate normal age/stage-related biological, psychological, and social changes leads to stagnation and psychosocial wheel spinning. The sense of an individual self is created early in life and it is the foundation of personality. However, not until adulthood does an individual fully develop a sense of a life cycle.

Erikson (1959), for example, identifies eight stages in the individual life cycle. Each stage of human growth is characterized by major developmental tasks of individual choice preferences regarding environmental demands and relational patterns, e.g., the choice of basic trust in the period covering the first year of life; autonomy and control, ages 1 to 3; initiative and doing, ages 4 to 6; industry and skill development, ages 6 to 12; identity and social solidarity, ages 12 to 20; intimacy versus isolation and generativity versus stagnation in mid-adulthood; and integrity versus despair in old age.

The last stage of life is necessarily the most difficult to deal with because it presupposes successful negotiation of previous developmental tasks. The choices reflecting integrity suggest a reconciliation and a synthesis of meaning in a final combination of all aspects of selfhood. Despair is characterized by a sense of incompleteness and malingering sorrow. The individual needs the cooperation of the social environment in order to sense the meaningfulness and purposefulness of life. Integration is not a sullen, isolated choice. Verwoerdt (1981) observes that

> it is no exaggeration to say that the social environment up until now has been less than conducive toward successful completion of the ultimate task in life: the final integration of one's self and of all past selves in the present self. Biological and social environmental hazards contribute to a great number of crises and failures (p. 14).

Neugarten (1976) notes in a similar view that the life cycle must mesh historical time, chronological time, and social time in order to preserve the individual's current and projected identity and integrity.

When an individual fails to attain integrity, a unique type of hopelessness and helplessness prevails. There is a loss of connection to others and a disorientation of values. Anomie, or a sense of disconnection from the valued mainstream of society, is closely linked to many emotional disorders, including suicide. If the aged are disconnected, how did they get that way and what can be done?

The family system functions as a conduit for age- and stage-related transitions along the developing life cycle. Stress in families is highest at the transition points from one stage to the next. Symptoms of dysfunction are most likely to appear when there is an interruption or dislocation in the unfolding family life cycle (Hadley, Jacob, Milliones, Caplain, & Spitz, 1974). One or more of the family members at those points of change may seek outside professional advice. Usually the members of the middle-aged or bridge generation are the ones who directly search for professional help; other members may express their need in less direct ways. The urgency of family derailment is described in phrases like "we must do something about Dad" or "Mom can't stay in that apartment alone any longer" or "I just don't know what I'd do if Dad dies."

Developmental theory may be useful in order to explain the cries for help along the family life cycle, but the important statistic for professionals in evaluating and treating suffering in the stages of life is N=1. One of one individual grows, develops, changes, and dies. One of one family will have difficulties with life transitions and have older members with unmet mental health needs. One of one will look to professionals for help in meeting the demands of developmental change at some point in the suffering.

Unfortunately, a number of factors in American society conspire to make the final stage of the life cycle relatively meaningless for too many older persons and their families. Weinberg (1979, 1981), a geriatric psychiatrist, suggests that at least three sources of suffering influence mental health and adjustment in later life: reality, cultural bias, and intrapersonal conflicts. The following remarks are indebted to Weinberg's insight and formulation of potential problem areas.

Reality

The strongest force in human suffering, not surprisingly, is reality. Reality is a source of human discomfort because the reality of later life is often characterized by real loss, real illness, and real isolation. Loss, as well as the fear of loss, both internal and external, is a predominant theme in the emotional life of older persons. Butler and Lewis (1973) point out that the elderly are confronted by multiple losses occurring simultaneously or at least in rapid succession, such as loss of a work role; economic loss; loss of significant others such as spouses, siblings, and peers; loss of self-esteem, status, and prestige; loss of health and energy; and actual physical loss of brain cells, including motor, memory, and sensory abilities. There is an "almost phobic dislike of aging in our society . . . the behavioral sciences had . . . mirrored societal attitudes by presenting old age as a grim litany of physical and emotional ills" (Butler & Lewis, 1973, p. 17).

Physical illness in later life is very real. It appears with greater frequency and greater complexity; recovery is typically slower. Savitsky and Sharkey (1972) note that a person may be said to be aging until there is a serious breakdown in functioning. Cumulative impairments in physical, emotional, and social skills reach a point of dysfunction and the person becomes "aged."

Neugarten (1979), a pioneer in aging research, states that psychological change is continuous throughout the life cycle, and individuals have a mental clock telling them where they are and whether they are on time. Individual biological aspects may or may not be in time with the psychological expectations. The mind/body systems move at different rates as biological clocks for certain organ systems begin to tick away. The biological, psychological, and social aspects of aging within a given individual may lack synchronization. The mind and body may be changing at drastically different rates. It is as if the system of the aging self gets out of step, resulting in an awkwardness making the individual and others around uncomfortable and uncertain. Physical desires may outstrip the body's capacity to respond. The mind may be intact but vision and hearing are impaired or lost. A variety of insults are experienced by the mind, body, or both. Fear of the untimely deaths of supportive friends, spouses, or relatives; fear of incapacitating illness; fear of not dying soon enough; fear of being the last survivor; and fear of not fitting in stalk the thoughts of many older persons. The diminished mastery, the losses, and the loss of synchronization of mind/body systems converge to make growing old in America a crisis in slow motion.

Cultural Bias

Cultural biases and social determinants are a substantial source of suffering at all stages of the life cycle. Whereas reality provides the context of human behavior, the sociocultural structures, expressed in value systems, provide the ideological interpretation of human behavior. In American culture, the old elicit strong emotional currents in all of us. Aging is generally viewed as decline, with little redeeming personal or social value. Aged persons frequently are perceived as unattractive, with rather unsatisfactory lives (Harris & Associates, 1975). The process of enculturation prepares our children to internalize these prejudices so that a system of automatic depreciation is built into later life. Cultural values have a significant impact on the elderly individual's sense of self-worth and avenues to the mainstream.

Our culture, according to some authors, has chosen to invest in the future. The elderly have no future, so they are not a good investment. Our elderly look to the past in a society that is future-oriented. Kluckhohn (1953), an anthropologist, described the three types of personality valued by a culture. Weinberg (1979) related these preferred classes to the social disenfranchisement that the elderly are experiencing. The three types are the "being," with a *now* focus on impulses, feelings, and satisfactions of the moment; the "being-in-becoming," most preoccupied with inner development and an emphasis on potential actualization of individual personality; and the "doing," the action-oriented person who is achievement-oriented and does. Doing—getting things done—is the most highly regarded mature personality expression. America's younger generation may be more focused on the now, but "doing" is still the most valued style. Whether this attitude will prevail remains to be seen.

For the moment, the older persons' loss of productivity is viewed in literal terms. A work role provides a person with a valued identity, a way to do, a way to discharge biological and psychic energy in meaningful and valued patterns of behavior. The elderly, forced into retirement, are devalued because they don't do. Our emphasis on the future and on productivity produces two classes of biases influencing later-life adjustment and self-esteem in significant ways.

Intrapersonal Conflicts

Intrapersonal struggles with the issues of integrity, dependency, and social connection often are major sources of suffering for older individuals as well as their families. The aging individual must accept his or her life as worthwhile, meaningful, and appropriate. If the individual does not resolve the final conflicts of integrity, then despair, depression, and bitterness result. Resolution of conflict implies some sense of competence. Effective integration and adjustment to one's life environment requires an intact ability to manipulate, to control, and finally to master the environment. Mastery in this sense results from the efforts of an effective problem-solving self successfully negotiating the biological, social, and psychological transitions inherent in the life cycle of development. White (1959) suggests that competence is the key ingredient in successful adjustment.

Goldfarb (1974) observes that competent or masterful older persons are able to gain gratification and discharge energy in meaningful patterns so as to maintain self-esteem, confidence, purposefulness, personal identity, and social role in spite of the losses accompanying the aging process (p. 823). An individual ego structure must mediate and integrate external and internal information. The ego, in many senses, is the problem-solving self, which maintains an appropriate balance between these sources of stimuli as the person negotiates development. Older persons, for a variety of causes, may begin to exclude too much external stimuli. Engagement is a complicated act involving perception and motivation. It is the point of contact between an individual and the environment. The tendency of older persons to turn inward for whatever reason excludes too much environmental stimuli, leading to discontinuous transactions in the social milieu.

Some authors such as Schaie (1977–78) view inward turning as adaptive and characteristic of the final developmental stage of the problem-solving self. Schaie postulates that during the life span there is a transition from "what I should know" through "how should I use what I know" to "why should I know." Schaie believes that the adult cognitive structure in old age may reach an overload demanding simplification. Cognitive energies evolve from a directive focus on acquisition in childhood and adolescents, to achievement in young adult life, to expectation and responsibility in middle age, and to reintegration in old age. The withdrawal of older persons, according to Schaie, may be a function of selective attention to certain environmental stimuli that have meaning and purpose within the immediate life stage situation or within a cosmic interest. Other areas of the environment may tend to be ignored. Consequently, selective intensity may be misinterpreted as disengagement.

Weinberg (1979) believes that exclusion of stimuli is a defense mechanism of an ego or self that is being threatened by a loss of roles and goals on all sides of the living process. Older persons do appear to be more inner focused; however, it may be more a matter of retreat than withdrawal. Families misinterpret and are stressed by withdrawal, often overreacting with extremes of social attentiveness and activity.

Appropriate adjustment within an environmental context is a common measure of mental health. There must be a healthy balance between the external and internal, or the individual is viewed as out of touch with the social milieu. The relative balance for each individual must be specifically and situationally understood, or intrapersonal conflicts will overwhelm the problem-solving self. However, as Williams (1972) observes, "there is a danger in simplifying mental illness as suffering and mental health as happiness" (p. 4). Mental health is more than the absence of mental illness. Many of the sources of intrapersonal suffering are developmental conditions or crises, not direct causes of mental illness. As Blau (1981) notes, "the cornerstones of an integrated personality are laid down in childhood, the struggle to achieve and sustain ego functions extend over a person's entire lifetime" (p. 133). The aged are not excused from responsibility for mental health, but they may need special support from their families in order to maintain their own health.

Most definitions of mental health outline signposts indicating whether a person has been able to negotiate the developmental tasks successfully. Jahoda (1958), for example, identifies six aspects of positive mental health—(1) a positive self-attitude, (2) growth and self-actualization, (3) integration of the personality, (4) autonomy, (5) reality perception, and (6) environmental mastery—as indicative of appropriate adjustment or balance between intrapersonal developmental challenges and environmental demands. A healthy personality must have the ability to love and relate to the social group, the ability to work and be productive (Freud, 1949). Maslow (1954) adds that a person must derive a sense of satisfaction and self-actualization from the process of growth and development. Issues concerning relating, identity, and control then become the areas of conflict for families as they and the older person attempt to make sense of the changes that come with growing older.

Both proponents and critics of the "disengagement theory" agree that the family remains the focus of social interaction for aging persons (Troll, 1971). Disengagement, when it occurs, is not always by choice. Older persons may disconnect from nonsatisfying, overdemanding social contracts but hold on to the family no matter what (Brown, 1974). Elderly persons and families who have invested in each other during a lifetime have many options. Elderly persons who have been noncaring and nongiving have fewer ties that bind and carry them through to the final life stage (Sussman, 1976).

It appears that the most vulnerable older person has a history of limited affective or emotional investment, lives in a narrow information stream, has functioned in highly specialized social roles, and has very high personal expectations in relation to his or her self-concept (Birren & Renner, 1980). It appears also that an individual's aging experience is mitigated by the characteristics of the family support system (Stuart & Snope, 1981).

Aging and Mental Health

Aging and mental health are arbitrarily defined by social groups. The definition of aging, as Butler and Lewis (1973) note, is merely a social convenience. The choice of age 65 to mark middle from old age was borrowed from the social policies of Bismark and Germany in the 1880s. This marker has functioned as a means of determining retirement or eligibility for a variety of services. Its arbitrary nature is evident in the past congressional action to change the demarcation to age 70 or do away with markers completely. Even gerontologists are struggling with the concept; they talk of the young-old (65-74 years) and old-old (75+ years).

Biological definitions of aging vary from social policies. They are narrow, typically stressing decline of functions. For example, Comfort (1956) stated that "senescence is a change in the behavior of the organism with age which leads to a decreased power of survival" (p. 190). Similarly, Handler (1960) wrote that "aging is the deterioration of a mature organism resulting from time-dependent, essentially irreversible changes intrinsic to all members . . . thereby increasing the possibility of death" (p. 200).

Recently, Birren and Renner (1977) offered a broader biologically based definition that allows for change and growth while acknowledging decline. "Aging refers to the regular changes that occur in mature genetically representative organisms living under representative environmental conditions as they advance in chronological age" (p. 4).

Current definitions of aging emphasize that age itself is not equivalent to an independent stage in the life cycle. Each life of each aging person is a singular experience. The commonalities, particularly the negative aspects, are more a matter of stereotyping and prejudice than fact. The facts are that aging occurs at three interrelated levels: the biological, the psychological, and the social. Biological aging refers to those changes in the structure and function of body organs and systems that occur during the life of an organism.

While biological aging is more often assumed to play the primary role in causing changes in behavior, biological factors alone cannot explain many major changes in behavior in the mature adult years. Psychological aging refers to changes in adaptive behavior due to increased experiences and changes in one's perception and identification of one's self as a result of biological or psychological processes. Social aging includes changes in norms, expectations, social status, and social roles available to a person over the course of a life span. A reductionist's view of aging tends to emphasize biological factors only. The biological approach ignores the sociocultural determinants of age-associated behavior and prevents differentiation of changes intrinsic to the aging process and those merely associated with old age due to social and environmental influences.

Many of the attitudes toward aging that influence later-life adjustments are shaped by prejudice and negative social expectations. Age prejudice or "age-ism" (Butler, 1974) is influenced by ideas concerning arbitrary age limits for certain behaviors.

Arbitrary age limits established for behavior (Troll & Nowak, 1976) could be titled *age restrictiveness;* that is to say, a span of years within which certain behaviors are considered appropriate is agreed upon and valued. When behavior occurs outside that span, it is labeled inappropriate and reacted to negatively. American humor ofter reveals discomfort with behaviors that are age-restrictive. "You shouldn't be doing/thinking that at your age." Unfortunately, our age limits for appropriate behavior were culturally established before people began living so long. Chronological age is a poor yardstick of appropriate behavior; norms are in a state of flux.

Another misconception supporting ageism is *age distortion.* In general, the greatest distortions seem to be for two extreme age groups, adolescence and old age (it is interesting to note that both of these groups are disenfranchised by our society, and the developmental stage is merely endured). We expect adolescence to be a stormy time of irresponsibility and self-centeredness. The aged are expected to be inactive, rigid, and conservative. This preoccupation that people *act their age* within severely narrow limits restricts potential behaviors for all groups. Most typically, adolescence is considered a scourge and old age, a disease. Old age is not a disease, although the aging process may make an individual more susceptible to disease (Cohen, 1974). Old age is a challenge in adjustment and coping with the changes that living brings. The physical aspects of aging are insignificant in comparison to the social and psychological aspects. If the aged weaken their ties with reality, perhaps it is because the reality represented for them is too painful to bear.

Until recent times, only the affluent and gifted have been given dispensation to grow old with any real sense of fulfillment and mastery. The higher mental illness rates among the aged become more understandable if we view the dual hazards of enforced inactivity and isolation that typify growing older in America and that loosen ties to the mainstream milieu.

The mental health needs growing from the sources of suffering are truly significant. Age restrictiveness and age distortions further contribute to these hazardous conditions. Lowenthal, Berkman, and associates reported in 1967 that 30 percent of the aged population suffered from moderate to severe psychiatric problems; 10 percent of these individuals were reported to need hospitalization. Kramer (1975, 1976) estimated that at this level of need a total of 2,405,300 individuals would need psychiatric care in 1980. The needs are dramatically revealed in Pfeiffer's (1977) report indicating that people over the age of 65 accounted for nearly 32 percent of all the suicides in the United States in 1970. Despite the extent of psychiatric impairments, older persons generally receive fewer mental health services than any other age group and evidence generally low utilization of psychiatric outpatient services (Gurland, Kuriansky, Sharpe, Simon, Stiller, & Birkett, 1977–78). Older persons are not likely to receive help for their psychiatric problems; admission to a nursing home is the more common solution (Birren & Renner, 1980).

Depression, loneliness, grief, anxiety, and stress are not unique to the aged. These emotions are part of the human condition, but why are these emotional reactions heightened in the final stage of growth? Rosow (1974) believes that the aged lack role clarity because of a weak socialization process of our society for old age.

In all cliches, stereotypes, and social myths, there are seeds of truth. Some of the negative views regarding old age grow from our confusion, misunderstanding, and lack of a knowledge base and experience with aging. Others may be completely inaccurate or biased, reflecting fear, prejudice, and, at times, outright hostility. Their hands are so cold, their faces so wrinkled, and their gait so uncertain that the prognosis frightens even the strongest of us. The loss of hearing, vision, memory, and physical mobility may be accepted especially if alleviated by changes in life style and expectations, but chronic debilitating illness is a specter hovering over all of us (Shahady, Cassata, & Cogswell, 1980). If the older person is aging or aged, so are other persons within the family. The slip from *senior* to *senile* is insidious and feared. The elderly experience human feelings that are both unique and yet similar to those experienced by all. Many older persons do live productively within a family system in the community and they are flexible and responsive to change. Other older persons merely fulfill society's prophecies. Fortunately, a new value system is emerging, one that calls for new roles for the elderly, expanded support systems, and new relationships among education, work, and leisure. Opportunities for older persons to continue education, pursue hobbies, and participate in the mainstream of their society are expanding, and new family-sensitive treatment modalities are evolving.

Mental Health of the Aged within a Family Context

In general, four identifiable areas of mental health needs are expressed by older persons within the family milieu. Older persons have a need: (1) to sense belonging; (2) to integrate past, present, and future life experiences; (3) to adapt or adjust to changing demands from both internal and external sources; and (4) to be supported in managing final life transitions in preparation for death. The family context affecting successful resolution of these needs is diverse and complex. Family functioning has changed as a result of significant changes in formal family organization and changes in the number, age, and composition of the generations. Similarly, the shortage of helping professionals coupled paradoxically with the bureaucratization of many family support activities, in the form of public services, is creating a maze of uncertainty and confusion over who should do what for whom. Treas (1979) argues that the evolution of public service bureaucracies to provide services to aging individuals has occasioned both greater problems and greater potential for intergenerational families.

The intersecting trends of social changes, demographic changes, and public service changes are drastically affecting the context of interaction within families and ultimately the satisfaction of the needs of the members. The family has been the primary and preferred social institution to deal with physical, social, and economic problems of older members (Bengston & Treas, 1980, p. 400). However, as our culture suffers the "future shock" of a nation growing old, families are struggling on a practical level to incorporate changes in essential areas of their socialization and valuing processes.

Most personality theorists agree that the mental health needs of an individual are dependent upon a positive self-concept formed and strengthened through social interaction. The family milieu is the first and perhaps the most pervasive context of continual socialization in our culture (Turner, 1962). Neugarten (1976) observes that the significant turning points in life—graduation, marriage, birth of children, career achievement, and the like—are "punctuation marks along the life cycle" that bring about changes in self-concept. New social roles are incorporated and, accordingly, they are the precipitants of new adaptations. These developmental challenges along with those of later life are usually faced within the context of family relationships (Birren & Renner, 1980). Most frequently in typical family functioning, there is an intergenerational connection and interdependent futures. Families are the first link in caring for older persons. However, important demographic and sociological trends are significantly impacting the family's abilities to carry out its natural support functions.

Demographic and Sociological Trends

The shifting age structure of Americans needing public services is a point of intense concern, labeled the "geriatric imperative" by some authors. There are more older people in need and they are growing older in terms of model age

Figure 1–1 United States Population and Elderly Percentages for Selected Years

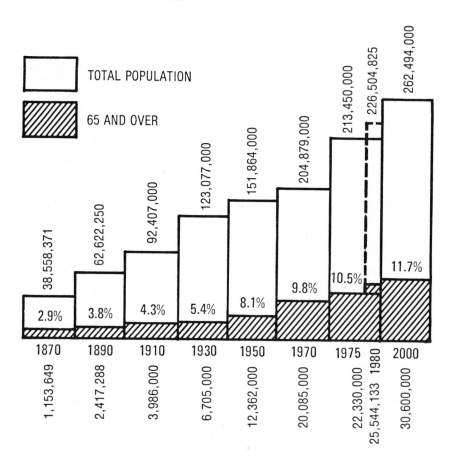

Note: Since starting this book, we have been advised by Herman Brotman that the total 1980 population figures for all ages have increased faster than 1980 projected figures. In addition to all age projections from 222,769,000 to 226,504,825, the over-65 age group increased from a projected 24,523,000 to 25,544,133. The figures reflect a .227 percent increase in the population rate for the over-65, from 11.0 percent to 11.227 percent. This projection must also be considered in the year 2000 projections. The population increase is based on the first count of the 1980 census plus recent data on life expectancy showing an increase in the upper ages due primarily to decreasing death rates from heart disease.

Source: U.S. Department of Commerce, Bureau of the Census, *Historical Statistics of the United States: Colonial Times to 1970* (Washington, D.C.: Government Printing Office, 1975), pp. 10 and 15. The figures for 1975 and 2000 are projections based on Brotman's research. For details, see Herman B. Brotman "Population Projections," *Gerontologist,* 1977, *17,* 203–209.

groups. Figure 1–1 illustrates the changing absolute numbers of older persons and the proportions of aged within the total population. Moreover, the older population is growing at a faster rate than other age classes, as a result of increasing life expectancy.

Demographers report that, from 1900 to 1970, life expectancy at birth increased from 47 to 73 years, a gain of 55 percent, or 26 years. Life expectancy refers to the average remaining years of life for an individual at a particular age. Life expectancy is differentiated from life span. Life span refers to the possible biological length of life (Hauser, 1976). Life expectancy has increased significantly, but the human life span has increased very little and is predicted to peak at about 85 years of age (Fries, 1980). There are more people today over the age of 65, but the human life span actually has not increased. More people are merely living out their natural life.

Brotman (1977) reports that, between the years 1975 and 2000, "the 55–64 age group will increase by 16%, the 65–74 group by 23% and the most vulnerable, the 75+ by 60%" (p. 209). A definite trend toward shorter age spans between generations is evident with more older persons having "old" children (Brody, 1966). There has been an increase in the number of four-generation families (Townsend, 1966) and a trend for three generations to develop within a time period that formerly produced two generations (Chilman, 1966). The impact of these trends on the family as a support system has only recently been acknowledged (Shanas & Hauser, 1974; Treas, 1977). The elderly and their aging family will be quickly stratified into age groups of younger aged, older aged, and, perhaps, middle aged. Brody (1966) notes that the aged, far from being homogeneous, will be confronted with problems unique to each age strata and with problems impinging on the other age groups. Increasingly, an aging parent is very old. The older age stratum (75+) is associated with greater declines in physical health and functional capacities that will inevitably tax the family support system, which is aging itself (Bengston & Treas, 1980). The longevity as well as the absolute numbers of the old will generate an unusual demand on health-related services, perhaps overwhelming the family as well. As 68-year-old daughters are attempting to care for 89-year-old mothers, the mismatch in care needs becomes more evident.

The existing disparity between the numbers of older women compared to older men will also continue to increase. In 1975, there were 144 women per 100 men over the age 65. By the year 2000, the ratio will be 154:100. For individuals aged 75+, the ratio is 171:100 and will be 191:100 by the year 2000 (Brotman, 1977, p. 209).

The configuration of kin networks is changing as well. An individual who will be 70 years old in the year 2000 is likely to average 1.4 siblings, 3.2 children, and 6.1 grandchildren. The immediate kin network would include 11.68 members; if spouses are counted, the network would total approximately

16 members. This network will decrease one-fourth for the next generations. In the year 2025 an individual will have 2.2 siblings, 1.9 children, and 4 grandchildren, for a total of 8.1 persons in the kin network. Spouses would increase this count to approximately 12 members (U.S. Bureau of the Census, 1977). The family is aging as well as the nation. The dependency needs of the old-old will be increasing at a time when many adult children will be attempting to meet their own dependency needs.

As a result of diverse social changes, there is no typical American family today, as Table 1–1 clearly indicates. Even though the figures represent guesses, Census Bureau statistics do show that the traditional concept of a nuclear group with a mother, father, and two children is in a minority (Skolnick & Skolnick, 1977). The birthrate is the lowest in our history and the divorce rate the highest. The frequency of divorce and remarriage has contributed greatly to the diversity of relational patterns organized around the concept of family. The "blended" family, composed of a husband, wife, and children from previous marriages, is more common; stepparenting has created new "extended families" of ex-spouses, associated grandparents, children, and stepsiblings (Goldenberg & Goldenberg, 1980, p. 11). The nature of relationships between generations in "blended" and new "extended families" is still evolving; no appropriate role models exist to guide individuals in enacting new family support patterns.

There is even current disagreement over what entity constitutes a family. Generally, modern society still tends to define the structure of a family in terms of its functions. Sussman (1976, p. 244) suggests a two-part definition. The first component is a "living together" group of individuals—which includes sanctioned or unsanctioned variant family forms involved in domestic functions and emotional and sexual cohabitation. This aspect of defining family recognizes that commitment, attachment, and emotional exchange and reinforcement are basic processes for individual and group survival. The second component is the conjugal family form consisting of "a nucleus of spouses and their offspring surrounded by a fringe of relatives" (Linton, 1936, p. 159); this best fits traditional social concepts of family. In this form, there is usually legitimization and religious sanction of marriage contracts, which circumscribe the rights and responsibilities of those involved. The official sanctioning also prescribes the linkage of an individual within a nuclear family to extended kin living some distance away.

Current linkages for the aged and their families often result in "intimacy at a distance" (Rosenmayr & Kockeis, 1963); psychosocial support, especially along generational lines; and assistance in domestic and economic functions (Sussman, 1965). The popularly held belief in modern society that because older people typically do not reside with the conjugal family, they are alienated from the family, is still being debated. Blau (1981) argues that "intimacy at a

Table 1-1 Variations in Family Pattern Types

FAMILY TYPE	CHARACTERISTICS	ESTIMATED PERCENT DISTRIBUTION IN U.S.
1. Nuclear family	Husband, wife & children living in common household	37
2. Nuclear aged	Husband & wife alone	11
3. Blended nuclear family	Husband, wife and usually children from previous marriage living in common household	11
4. Single Parent family	One parent household as a result of divorce, death, or never married	12
5. Extended family	Husband, wife, children plus grandparents, uncles aunts, etc. Three generations living in close proximity and reciprocal exchanges of goods, services and resources	4
6. Single members	Single, separated, widowed or divorced adults living alone	19
7. Experimental and emerging forms		
Commune	Men, women, & children together collectively sharing labor, property, production & services	
Common law	Families of choice - man, woman, and perhaps natural offspring legally sanctioned in some states in a given period of time	
Co-Habitation	A variant of common law with adults sharing living arrangements and providing mutual support. Usually no child.	6
		100

Source: Percent distributions based on Marvin B. Sussman, The Family Life of Old People. In R.H. Binstock & E. Shanas (Eds.), *Handbook of Aging and The Social Sciences,* 1976.

distance'' is merely a euphemism for pseudointimacy between generations and serves only to obfuscate the actual alienation.

In most cases, patterns of family relating are fairly constant. Gaitz (1978) points out that the elderly accept physical and financial assistance from adult children and adult children gradually assume a more caretaking role characterized by "filial maturity." Filial maturity (Blenkner, 1965) involves accepting responsibility for the aging parents' dependency needs in a positive manner. In families with a history of conflict, the dependency requests of aging parents precipitate conflicts. Generally the research shows that family support is flowing in both directions, based on need, resources, and opportunity (Riley, 1976). Many older persons give adult children more than they receive (Rosenfeld, 1978). A living pattern has emerged whereby 75 percent of old people have children residing within a 30-minute travel time and 90 percent report having seen one or more adult child within a month (Shanas, 1968). The relative satisfaction of these contacts remains uncertain and undocumented.

The historical stereotyping of older people living under the same roof within an extended family is also generally untrue. Dahlin (1980) reports that at the turn of the century most old people were the heads of households, not dependents in the homes of their children or grandchildren. Grown children at times lived with their parents. In 1900, 42 percent of married old people lived in the same household with one or more of their unmarried children. By contrast, in 1970 only 10 percent lived with their children. The number of older persons living alone or with their spouses has risen from 20 percent in 1900 to 75 percent in 1975 (Dahlin, 1980, p. 105). The trend is for old people—couples or singles—to maintain their own household. Today, one in seven men over the age of 65 lives alone whereas nearly one-third of women over age 65 live alone (U.S. Department of Health, Education, and Welfare, 1978). In addition, 17 percent of the men over 65 are widowed. This figure rises to 30 percent at the age of 75 or over. For women, 54 percent over age 65 are widowed. In the over-75 age group, fully 70 percent are widowed. A further implication is that at age 65 there are four women to every three men, but at age 85 there are two women for every man (U.S. Department of Health, Education, and Welfare, 1978). Couples living together appear to have more social togetherness and fewer perceived problems. Single elderly persons, though, seem to exhibit more fear or anxieties, mostly derived from their inability to cope with the demands of daily living, and are more likely to be institutionalized (Stuart & Snope, 1981).

Family size has also changed dramatically. In 1860 the conjugal family size was 5.1; in 1960 it was 3.7. In 1980 it is projected to be even smaller. The spacing of children is affecting modern family structure. Childbearing years have been reduced and compressed so that the space between generations is narrower, ages of siblings closer, and number of siblings fewer.

The role of women has changed significantly over this century. More women work out of the home, with a working mother in 20 percent of families (Kuhn, 1980). Young working women with children expect their mothers to help with child caring and even household maintenance, an expectation strongly resented by some older persons (Cohler & Grunebaum, 1981). The proportion of women in the labor force has increased. By the year 2000, 57 to 60 percent of all women will be employed. Women traditionally have been the "kinkeeper," coordinating family transactions and initiating family support exchanges. Working women will not be able to provide the same degree of assistance to family transactions, including those with older members. For these reasons Treas (1977) cautions that "the current enthusiasm for family-based alternatives to institutionalized care for the aged must be tempered by realistic expectation of the willingness and ability of modern American women to provide continued services for aging kin" (p. 488).

The role of public service agencies in providing care and support has increased in recent years; however, the future is uncertain. Social assistance services in the areas of health, transportation and housing and other services necessary to the general welfare have mushroomed as a result of federal legislation. However, Sussman (1976) argues that the bureaucratization of support has merely supplemented, not surplanted, the families' role as caregivers. Older persons largely remain physically independent but psychologically dependent on their families despite the proliferation of public services. Families are still the preferred source of assistance especially in times of crisis (Hill, Foote, Aldous, Carlson, & MacDonald, 1970). Although it is popularly assumed that older persons are confined to nursing homes, psychiatric institutions, and homes for the aged, in fact only 4 percent live in nursing homes and 1 percent in all other types of institutions. In total, only 5 percent of the older population are placed out of their homes (Shanas, 1979a).

The majority of older persons live in their own homes in a familiar community. Even with the new forms of public services and assistance, families are still attending to their responsibilities. Studies of aging in every country consistently find that older persons who are isolated and lacking family and social support are often institutionalized even when not greatly incapacitated; studies also find that the bulk of services even in developed countries is performed by relatives (Little, 1980). An estimated 80 percent of all home health care is provided by families. Solidarity and affection remain part of the family function (Brody, 1980).

Character of Current Patterns of Family Support

The studies that have examined the character of family support report certain consistencies in caregiving roles. Families are caring for elderly members, at times at the expense of other important family relationships (Brody, 1977). Blau (1981, p. 49) observes that adult children experience significant conflicts in family priorities as they attempt to meet the demands of daily living and the needs of aging parents. The sense of family obligation is alive and well in the United States, but stress arises from attempts to meet responsibilities to spouses, children, and aging parents. Johnson and Bursk (1977) note, not surprisingly, that older parents rated the significance of relating to their adult children higher than adult children rate the significance of relating to their aging parents. Interpersonal conflicts and restrictions on adult childrens' privacy and freedom stress the caregiving relationship (Newman, 1976). As the "me" generation senses its own personal stresses of parenting, economic and vocational achievement, generativity, and intimacy, the stresses on the caregiving relationship are likely to continue.

Patterns of family caregiving based on observational data reveal that several categories of family support activities are evident in present-day caregiving. The services most frequently provided by family members are preparing meals, light housekeeping, administering or supervising medication, and assisting with personal grooming and hygiene. The most infrequently provided support activities are major home repairs, transportation, and constant supervision of a seriously impaired person (Frankfather, Smith & Caro, 1981). Generally, care requiring living-in precedes entrance to an institution (Shanas, 1979a). However, even after institutionalization, the family maintains ties. York and Calsyn (1977) report, for example, that the mean number of monthly family visits to older members in nursing homes was 12.

Recent data show another side of the family relating coin, as evidenced by Cohler and Grunebaum (1981) in a recent interview. They tell of a middle-aged Boston woman who works as a seamstress all week and for her parish on Sundays. Every Saturday, her daughter and family visit with the expectation that mother/grandmother will make lunch, visit, or go shopping. In four New England families studied, the older women resented the numerous phone calls, visits, and general dependencies of their grown daughters. Working women are turning to the grand generations for advice, physical resources, emotional support, and companionship as well as babysitting services. The full impact of this recent phenomenon on the individuals involved as well as the family structure clearly needs further exploration.

Some factors make caregiving patterns more stress resistive. These include a history of patterns of mutual aid and affection (Newman, 1976), a high degree of perceived support from other family members, and a gradual rather than sudden increase in the needs of the older person (Kerschner, 1980, p. 108).

Sussman (1979) reports that a majority of families would prefer some form of financial assistance in caring for an older member. Further analysis of the data revealed that the trend of desired financial support was voiced by families who had not yet experienced caring for a dependent older member. Conversely, families who had provided care desired greater availability of service supports. While these families recognized the benefits of financial aid, they were more realistically concerned with the development of services in the community, such as homemaking services, shopping, and transportation, that would ease the caregiving tasks. Similar findings were reported in a study by the U.S. General Accounting Office in 1976.

As the adult child becomes increasingly involved in providing support, the situation becomes more complex. Newman (1975) reports that when the disability of aging parents reaches a point of requiring extended care, only two alternatives are usually considered: moving the older person into a nursing home or into the home of a family member. Robinson and Thurnher (1979) conclude that adult children strive to delay institutionalization of the impaired elderly at considerable cost to themselves and their nuclear family. The poorer the health of the older person, the more likely they are to be found residing in the same household with adult children (Shanas, 1960). As dependencies increase, both the older parent and adult children are aware of the potential conflicts (Shanas, 1962). The stresses on the adaptive capacity of the family system, not the specific health problems of the older members, lead to a decline in the quality of family relating and the placement of the aged out of the home and into a long-term care institution (Kraus, Spasoff, Beattie, Holden, Lawson Rodenburg, & Woodcock, 1976).

Despite the stresses and excessive demands upon emotional and economic resources, the majority of the frail elderly are living in their own homes with support or in homes of family members (Shanas, 1979b). As individuals, the impaired elderly tend to avoid seeking help outside the family for a variety of reasons. Often the nature of the mental illness itself interferes with the process of seeking help (Cohen, 1976). Consequently, the problem-solving and decision-making processes are more likely to fall on the families' shoulders. Cognitive impairments, memory losses, and mental illness of older members continue to be extremely difficult burdens for families (Issacs, 1971). Little respite is available in the foreseeable future if new models of family assessment and care are not developed. The changing context of aging, mental health, and family patterns represents a dilemma in providing adequate and appropriate care to older persons. Bengston and Treas (1980) comment that "on the one hand family relationships are crucial in meeting predictable mental health needs; on the other hand, social change, professional shortages and demographic trends are drastically altering the traditionally prescribed roles and responsibilities of family groups" (p. 401).

Families remain the most important support system for older members. The older person is most likely to turn to the family first, then to friends and neighbors, and use public social services last (Shanas, 1979b). Ethnic groups show some variation in this pattern. Hispanics, for example, are more reluctant to turn to professionals for help (Valle & Mendoza, 1978); nonminority elderly, in general, are more likely than minority elders to seek professional help (Weeks & Cuellar, 1981).

Only a small percentage of older persons have no surviving children. The special problems of these individuals are being considered in a variety of ways. There is an increasing awareness that natural support systems should be facilitated and strengthened (Stanford, 1980). This natural support system may well include the filial function of responsibilities assumed by nieces, nephews, cousins, more functional siblings, or unrelated lifelong acquaintances and friends. Suggestions for promoting the development of natural or nonbureaucratic support include "surrogate families," neighborhood social networking, and cooperative groups such as Kuhn's (1980) "families of choice." The families of choice and surrogate families are described by Kuhn as intergenerational groups of nonrelated individuals who share resources, goals, values, and life styles over time and produce a network of mutual responding and support giving.

Consequently, the term *family* is itself changing to include a broad range of support alternatives. These changes have significant implications for public policy regarding family legislation and should be reflected upon before caregiving programs for older needy persons are implemented. Except for individuals who are extremely impaired, it is more cost-effective to maintain a family's older person in the community with a coordinated service package characterized by "surrogate" family support activities.

BRIEF REVIEW OF FAMILY TREATMENT APPROACHES

Since the 1950s, a number of behavioral sciences have focused on the family context of individual adjustment and mental health. The field of family therapy literally erupted in 1957 as a national meeting for family researchers coalesced upon the issues. It was as if the notion of family-oriented therapy suddenly became legitimate (Bowen, 1980). This period of development reflected the election of numerous theoretical postures and therapeutic modes. At least five clinical movements significantly influenced subsequent evolution of the field of family treatment: (1) psychoanalysis, (2) general systems theory, (3) research of schizophrenia, (4) marital counseling and child guidance, and (5) group therapy (Goldenberg & Goldenberg, 1980).

A brief review of these developments and when they evolved aids in our understanding current approaches to treatment within a family system. Psychoanalysis, as expressed by Freud and his followers, focused on individual intrapsychic conflicts and resolution. Ackerman (1958) elaborated and extended the psychoanalytic approach to include the role of family in conflict. Ackerman characterized the family as "a kind of carrier of elements predisposing to both mental illness and mental health" (p. 104). Treatment of the family involves intervention at several levels, the individual personality, the role adaptation of family members, and the behavior of the family as a social system. Disturbances within the individual unbalance the family's relational patterns. Accordingly, the family in which disturbance occurs must be helped to accommodate new experiences, to cultivate new complementary levels in family role relationships, to find avenues for the solution of conflict, to build a favorable self-image, to buttress critical forms of defense against anxiety, and to provide support for further creative development (Ackerman, 1966, pp. 90–91).

Minuchin (1974) and Bowen (1978) continued to differentiate family therapy from individual treatment orientations by applying general systems theory to the structures of family groups and the functions of individuals within these groups. Systems theory proposes that all living systems exist in a hierarchy. A system is a complex whole made of component parts in mutual interactive relationship to other parts. To understand the individual part, one must study the transactions that the part has with other components and to systems at other levels. Systems contain self-regulating processes, homeostatic mechanics, and feedback loops. The disturbed or needy individual family member is just one part of a subsystem in the family system that influences and is influenced by disturbing individuals. A systems model encompasses the flow and interactive nature of the biological, psychological, and sociological forces that impinge upon an individual and family.

During the mid-1950s, three lines of family research in the area of schizophrenia converged to illuminate the role of a disturbed family environment in the development of mental illness. Bateson, an anthropologist, and his associates perceived the relation of pathological communication within family relations to development and maintenance of deviant behavior of individual members. They introduced the now famous "double-bind" theory of contrasting simultaneous information exchange between family members as a precursor to disturbances in individual growth and development (Bateson, Jackson, Haley, & Weakland, 1956). At about the same time, Theodore Lidz (Lidz, Fleck, & Cornelison, 1965) was extending psychoanalytic concepts to the family, and Murray Bowen (1960) began to work with the vacillations of intimacy that tend to be characteristic of families of schizophrenics. These researchers, who focused on the relationships between family processes and the development of schizophrenia, laid the groundwork and provided the impetus for what became the field of family therapy (Goldstein & Rodnick, 1975).

The fields of marital counseling and child guidance were clinical forerunners of family therapy that helped to change the focus of interventions from individually oriented psychotherapies to conjoint therapeutic approaches and an emphasis on relationships with respect to child guidance. Healy introduced the aspect of multidisciplinary teams to assess both the child in conflict and the family (Goldenberg, 1973). The practice of utilizing teams of psychiatrists, social workers, clinical psychologists, and often an educator, became a tradition at guidance clinics. The collaborative approach among professionals persists in family therapy, and the team concept is an important thrust in treatment.

Group therapy and milieu therapy quickly demonstrated the effectiveness of small social groups in bringing about therapeutic changes and in many ways were the outgrowth of new emphasis upon systems theory. The goal of therapy shifted from changing an individual's personality, organization, and behavior to changing interaction patterns and family structures.

Some 20 years later, as the implications of the systems theory approach continue to permeate aspects of mental health services, a concept of family as a unit that endures across time and space is coming into focus. The family life cycle as a treatment format is proving to be a practical and effective means of helping people move from viewing conflicts and deficiencies as individual problems (Carter & McGoldrick, 1980).

Medalie (1978, 1979) suggests a breakdown of the family life cycle into seven steps, each with its particular developmental task. The first step is premarital and early marital bonding. Step two reflects the expectant couple. Birth of a child launches step three. Multiple children or parenting adolescents is step four. Middle age is marked by the departure of the last child from home; thus step five is achieved as the family completes its formative and expansion stages and moves into a period of contradiction, the empty nest or "child-free" stage. Step six is late adulthood, usually lasting two decades and characterized by retirement. Widowhood, death of spouse, and death of surviving spouse characterize step seven, the final step in the life cycle of a family.

Hill (1970) emphasized three generational aspects of families, with each stage of the family life cycle bringing about distinctive role complexes. Duvall (1977) observed that the family as a whole has developmental tasks, as well as interest in achievements of one individual. One generation is dependent upon and contributes to the successful negotiation by other family members. Minuchen (1974) described the idea of the family developmental stage as the key concept in family therapy from a systems view. The goal of therapeutic intervention with dysfunctional families is to restore the capacity to support members adequately in attaining a successful resolution of developmental changes (Terkelsen, 1980), while preserving the integrity and boundaries of the family system itself.

The family life cycle movement within the field of family therapy is obviously gaining momentum as mental health and later-life adjustment are viewed within the context of family. Unfortunately, at this time, few if any models of therapeutic aging are available to guide families of impaired elderly and professionals alike through the stages. An expanded model must be constructed. The geriatric imperative creates a sense of urgency to which we must quickly respond.

GENERAL CONTOURS OF THE NEW FAMILY-CENTERED INTERVENTION MODEL

The evident psychological distress of the aging process and its impact on families urgently demands an integrative life-span model to guide assessment, coordinate treatment and intervention, and bridge the gap between theory and practice. Families encounter a variety of clinical and academic disciplines in their search for help with aging issues; however, the perspective and emphasis of these disciplines vary widely. Families are often left with a sense of fragmentation, incompleteness of theories, and frustration with current mechanisms of service delivery. Consequently, the emerging field of family gerontology initially requires an integration of the various professional models.

Fortunately, vigorous expansion of the aging knowledge base within the last 20 years has created a climate for integrative models, as Neugarten (1980) concludes that "aging is in." Issues concerning the family cycle, the life cycle, and aging will preoccupy human service providers for the next several decades. Today's questions involve what fits together, what doesn't. Where are the research gaps? Where are the service gaps? Where are the theories to bridge the gaps?

A number of sociocultural trends are coalescing to create a favorable climate for integration. The natural evolution of individual disciplines is beginning to clarify areas of common concern and integrate information relevant to aging. Diversification within more highly evolved disciplines, coupled with a holistic attitude toward mind/body issues, is promoting intense interaction relative to understanding the aging process.

Increased identification of the needs of the aging population as well as expansion of the population itself has also created a challenge in integrating service delivery. Limitations of resources, time, intellectual energy, money, and people are forcing a review of possible duplication or overlap in professional efforts and services. This appears true on both a national policy/administration level and on the practical, clinical level. Advocacy groups including families of older members are insisting on practical and useful information from the professional community and integration of scientific information into a usable form. Butler (1980) acknowledges the importance of this necessary but productive tension between advocacy and science and outlines the value of ongoing dialogue.

The shortage of trained medical personnel itself requires more highly organized, integrated information with a clarification of roles and responsibilities. According to a Rand Corporation study (Kane, 1980), the increase in the nation's elderly, coupled with physician indifference to this segment of the population, has created a major shortage of geriatricians. Cooperation among supporting disciplines in meeting the physical and mental health needs of the elderly has moved from the level of preference to necessity.

A multidisciplinary conceptualization of psychological distress in aging is complicated by the number of variables impacting the aging person's well-being. Unique personality characteristics as well as the degree of individual adaptive capacity at any given time to a given environment further add to the complexity. The dynamic quality of age-related changes and subsequent difficulties in differentiating normal from pathological distresses add to conceptual difficulties. The complexity and multiplicity of aging demand ongoing integration of subsets of information and reintegration of all component variables individually and simultaneously *while* everything is changing. A general conceptualization then becomes an evolving conceptualization with integrative value only at a given time.

The need to understand psychological distress in aging becomes the challenge to develop an appropriate matrix for organizing relevant information from the range of disciplines contributing to the knowledge base. Three general areas are emerging as descriptive points for an integrated approach. These general grid areas are biology, psychology, and society/environment. A new definition of aging clearly outlines the interactive aspects of a biopsychosocial view—biological referring to life expectancy, psychological referring to the adaptive behavioral capacities of the individual, and social referring to the social roles of an individual with regard to the expectations of his group and society for someone of that age (Birren & Renner, 1977, p. 5).

Development of a comprehensive model that organizes biopsychosocial variables and subsequently translates this integrated information in a utilitarian form to family caregivers is truly the mental health challenge of the 1980s. It is time to move forward with a plan to help families understand the biology of aging, support the psychology of aging, and assist with social-environmental needs of their older members.

REFERENCES

Ackerman, N.W. *The psychodynamics of family life.* New York: Basic Books, 1958.

Ackerman, N.W. *Treating the troubled family.* New York: Basic Books, 1966.

Bateson, G., Jackson, D., Haley, J., & Weakland, J. Towards a theory of schizophrenia. *Behavioral Science*, 1956, *1*, 251–264.

Bengston, V.L., & Treas, J. The changing family context of mental health and aging. In J.E. Birren and R.B. Sloan (Eds.), *Handbook of mental health and aging*. Englewood Cliffs, N. J.: Prentice-Hall, 1980.

Birren, J.E., & Renner, V.J. Research on the psychology of aging: Principles and experimentation. In J.E. Birren & K.W. Schaie (Eds.), *Handbook of aging and the individual*. New York: Van Nostrand Reinhold, 1977.

Birren, J.E., & Renner, V.J. Concepts and issues of mental health and aging. In J.E. Birren & R.B. Sloan (Eds.), *Handbook of mental health and aging*. Englewood Cliffs, N.J.: Prentice-Hall, 1980.

Blau, Z.S. *Aging in a changing society*. New York: Franklin Watts, 1981.

Blenkner, M. Social work and family relationships in later life with some thoughts on filial maturity. In E. Shanas & G.F. Streib (Eds.), *Social structure and the family: Generational relations*. Englewood Cliffs, N.J.: Prentice-Hall, 1965.

Bowen, M. A family concept of schizophrenia. In D.D. Jackson (Ed.), *The etiology of schizophrenia*. New York: Basic Books, 1960.

Bowen, M. *Family therapy in clinical practice*. New York: Jason Aronson, 1978.

Bowen, M. Foreward. In E. Carter & M. McGoldrick (Eds.), *The family life cycle: A framework for family therapy*. New York: Gardner Press, 1980.

Brody, E.M. The aging family. *Gerontologist*, 1966, *6*, 201–206.

Brody, E.M. *Long-term care of older people: Needs and options*. New York: Human Sciences Press, 1977.

Brody, E.M. Prepared statement. In *Families: Aging and changing* (Commerce Publication No. 96–242). Hearing before the Select Committee on Aging, U.S. House of Representatives, 96th Congress, Second Session. Washington, D.C.: U.S. Government Printing Office, June 4, 1980.

Brotman, H.B. Population projections: Part I. Tomorrow's older population (to 2000). *Gerontologist*, 1977, *17*, 203–209.

Brown, A.S. Satisfying relationships for the elderly and their patterns of disengagement. *Gerontologist*, 1974, *14*, 258–262.

Butler, R.N. Successful aging and the role of the life review. *Journal of the American Geriatrics Society*, 1974, *22*, 529–535.

Butler, R.N. Wanted: Information about and for the aging (an interview with Robert N. Butler, M.D., director of the National Institute on Aging). *Bulletin of the American Society for Information Science*, 1978, *5* (1), 14.

Butler, R.N. The alliance of advocacy with science. *Gerontologist*, 1980, *20*, 154–161.

Butler, R.N., & Lewis, M.I. *Aging and mental health*. St. Louis: C.V. Mosley, 1973.

Carter, E.A., & McGoldrick, M. The family life cycle and family therapy: An overview. In E. Carter and M. McGoldrick (Eds.), *The family life cycle: A framework for family therapy*. New York: Gardner Press, 1980.

Chilman, C.S. *Population dynamics and poverty in the United States* (Welfare in Review, Vol. 4, No. 3, U.S. Department of Health, Education, and Welfare). Washington, D.C.: U.S. Government Printing Office, 1966.

Cohen, C. Techniques in teaching geriatric medicine. In W. Anderson & T.G. Judge (Eds.), *Geriatric medicine*. New York: Academic Press, 1974.

Cohen, G.D. Mental health services and the elderly: Needs and options. *American Journal of Psychiatry*, 1976, *133*, 65–68.

Cohler, B.J., & Grunebaum, H.U. *Mothers, grandmothers and daughters.* New York: Wiley & Sons, 1981.

Comfort, A. *The biology of senescence.* London: Routledge and Kegan Paul, 1956.

Dahlin, M. Perspectives on the family life of the elderly in 1900. *Gerontologist,* 1980, *20,* 99–107.

Duvall, E. *Marriage and family development* (5th ed.). New York: Lippencott, 1977.

Erikson, E.H. Identity and the life cycle. *Psychological issues.* New York: International Universities Press, 1959.

Frankfather, D.L., Smith, M.J. & Caro, F.G. *Family care of the elderly.* Lexington, Mass.: Lexington Books, 1981.

Freud, S. *An outline of psychoanalysis.* New York: Norton, 1949.

Fries, J.F. Aging, natural death and the compression of morbidity. *The New England Journal of Medicine,* 1980, *303* (3), 130–135.

Gaitz, C.M. Aged patients, their families and physicians. In G. Usdin & C.K. Hofling (Eds.), *Aging, the process and the people.* New York: Brunner-Mazel, 1978.

Goldenberg, H. *Contemporary clinical psychology.* Monterey, Calif.: Brooks/Cole, 1973.

Goldenberg, I., & Goldenberg, H. *Family therapy: An overview.* Belmont, Calif.: Wadsworth, 1980.

Goldfarb, A.V. Minor maladjustment in the aged. In S. Arieti and E.B. Brody (Eds.), *American handbook of psychiatry* (Vol. 3). New York: Basic Books, 1974.

Goldstein, M., & Rodnick, E. The family's contribution to the etiology of schizophrenia: Current status. *Schizophrenia Bulletin,* 1975, *14,* 263–273.

Gurland, B., Kuriansky, J., Sharpe, L., Simon, R., Stiller, P., & Birkett, P. The comprehensive assessment and referral evaluation (CARE): Rationale, development and reliability. *International Journal of Aging and Human Development,* 1977–78, *8,* 9–42.

Hadley, T.R., Jacob, T., Milliones, J., Caplain, J., & Spitz, D. The relationship between family developmental crisis and the appearance of symptoms in a family member. *Family Process,* 1974, *13,* 207–214.

Handler, P. Radiation and aging. In N.W. Shock (Ed.), *Aging.* Washington, D.C.: American Association for the Advancement of Science, 1960.

Harris, L., & Associates. *The myth and reality of aging in America.* Washington, D.C.: The National Council on Aging, 1975.

Hauser, P.M. Aging and worldwide population change. In R.H. Binstock & E. Shanas (Eds.), *Handbook of aging and the social sciences.* New York: Van Nostrand Reinhold, 1976.

Hill, R., Foote, N., Aldous, J., Carlson, R., & MacDonald, R. *Family development in three generations.* Cambridge: Schenkman, 1970.

Issacs, B. Geriatrics patients: Do their families care? *British Medical Journal,* 1971, *4,* 282–286.

Jahoda, M. *Current concepts of positive mental health.* New York: Basic Books, 1958.

Johnson, E.S., & Bursk, B.J. Relationships between the elderly and their adult children. *Gerontologist,* 1977, *17,* 90–96.

Kalish, R.A., & Knudtson, F.W. Attachment versus disengagement: A life-span conceptualization. *Human Development,* 1976, *19,* 171–181.

Kane, R.L. Increase in nation's elderly seen creating shortage of geriatricians (Rand Corporation study). *American Medical News,* 1980, *27,* 3.

Kerschner, P. Family support systems and the aging: A policy report. In *Families: Aging and changing* (Commerce Publication No. 96–242). Hearing before the Select Committee on Aging,

U.S. House of Representatives, 96th Congress, Second Session. Washington, D.C.: U.S. Government Printing Office, June 4, 1980.

Klerman, G.L. Prepared statement. In *Aging and mental health: Overcoming barriers to service* (Commerce Publication No. 67-899-0). Hearing before the Special Committee on Aging, Part 2, U.S. Senate, 96th Congress, Second Session. Washington, D.C.: Government Printing Office, May 22, 1980.

Kluckhohn, C. Dominant and variant value orientations. In C. Kluckhohn & H. Murray (Eds.), *Personality of nature, society and culture.* New York: Alfred A. Knopf, 1953.

Kohlberg, L. Development of moral character and moral ideology. In M. Hoffman and L. Hoffman (Eds.), *Review of child development.* New York: Russell Sage Foundation, 1964.

Kohlberg, L. *Stages in the development of moral thought and action.* New York: Holt, Rinehart & Winston, 1969.

Kohlberg, L. Continuities in childhood and adult moral development revisited. In P. Baltes and K. Schaie (Eds.), *Life span developmental psychology: Personality and socialization.* New York: Academic Press, 1973.

Kramer, M. *Psychiatric services and the changing institutional scene.* Paper presented at the President's Biomedical Research Panel. Unpublished manuscript, November 25, 1975.

Kramer, M. Issues in the development of statistical and epidemeological data for mental health services research. *Psychological Medicine,* 1976, *6,* 185-215.

Kraus, A.S., Spasoff, R.A., Beattie, E.J., Holden, D.E., Lawson, J.S., Rodenburg, M., & Woodcock, G.M. Elderly applicants to long-term care institutions: The application process: placement and care needs. *Journal of the American Geriatrics Society,* 1976, *24,* 165-172.

Kuhn, M. Prepared statement. In *Families: Aging and changing* (Commercial Publication No. 96-242). Testimony before the Select Committee on Aging, U.S. House of Representatives, 96th Congress, Second Session. Washington, D.C.: U.S. Government Printing Office, June 4, 1980.

Lidz, T., Fleck, S., & Cornelison, A. *Schizophrenia and the family.* New York: International Universities Press, 1965.

Linton, R.L. *The study of man.* New York: Appleton-Century-Crofts, 1936.

Little, V.C. Assessing the needs of the elderly: State of the art. *International Journal of Aging and Human Development,* 1980, *11,* 65-76.

Lowenthal, M.F., Berkman, P.L., & associates. *Aging and mental disorders in San Francisco: A social psychiatric study.* San Francisco: Josey-Bass, 1967.

Maslow, A.H. *Motivation and personality.* New York: Harper and Row, 1954.

Medalie, J.H. (Ed.). *Family medicine: Principles and applications.* Baltimore: Williams & Wilkins, 1978.

Medalie, J.H. The family life cycle and its implications for family practice. *Journal of Family Practice,* 1979, *9,* 47-56.

Minuchin, S. *Families and family therapy.* Cambridge: Harvard University Press, 1974.

Neugarten, B.L. Adaptation and the life cycle. *The Counseling Psychologist,* 1976, *6,* 16-20.

Neugarten, B.L. Time, age and the life cycle. *American Journal of Psychiatry,* 1979, *136,* 887-894.

Neugarten, B.L. Acting one's age: New rules for old. *Psychology Today,* April, 1980, 66-80.

Neugarten, B.L., & Hagestad, G.O. Age and the life course. In R.H. Binstock and E.L. Shanas (Eds.), *Handbook of aging and the social sciences.* New York: Van Nostrand Reinhold, 1976.

Newman, S. *Housing adjustment of older people: A report of findings from the first phase.* Ann Arbor: University of Michigan, Institute for Social Research, 1975.

Newman, S. *Housing adjustment of older people: A report of findings from the second phase.* Ann Arbor: University of Michigan, Institute for Social Research, 1976.

Pfeiffer, E. Psychopathology and social pathology. In J.E. Birren & K.W. Schaie (Eds.), *Handbook of the psychology of aging.* New York: Van Nostrand Reinhold, 1977.

Piaget, J. *The construction of reality in the child.* New York: Basic Books, 1954.

Piaget, J. *The origins of intelligence in children.* New York: International Universities Press, 1963.

Piaget, J. Intellectual evolution from adolescence to adulthood. *Human Development,* 1972, *15* (1), 1–12.

Redick, R.W., & Taube, C.A. Demography and mental health care of the aged. In J.E. Birren & R.B. Sloan (Eds.), *Handbook of mental health & aging.* Englewood Cliffs, NJ: Prentice-Hall, 1980.

Riley, M.V. Social gerontology and the age stratification of society. In B. Hess (Ed.), *Growing old in America.* New Brunswick, N.J.: Transaction Books, 1976.

Robinson, B., & Thurnher, M. Taking care of aged parents: A family cycle transition. *Gerontologist,* 1979, *19,* 586–593.

Rosenfeld, A.H. *New views on older lives. A sampler of NIMH sponsored research and service programs* (U.S. Department of Health, Education, and Welfare Publication No. ADM 78-687). Rockville, Md.: U.S. Department of Health, Education, and Welfare, National Institute of Mental Health, 1978.

Rosenmayr, L., & Kockeis, E. Propositions for a sociological theory of aging and the family. *International Social Science Journal,* 1963, *15,* 410–426.

Rosow, I. *Socialization to old age.* Berkeley: University of California Press, 1974.

Savitsky, E., & Sharkey, H. The geriatric patient and his family: A study of family interaction in the aged. *Journal of Geriatric Psychiatry,* 1972, *5,* 3–19.

Schaie, K.W. Toward a stage theory of adult cognitive development. *Journal of Aging and Human Development,* 1977–78, *8* (2), 129–137.

Shahady, E.J., Cassata, D.M., & Cogswell, B.E. The "family" in family practice. *Family Medicine Teacher,* 1980, *12,* 4.

Shanas, E. Family responsibility and the health of older people. *Journal of Gerontology,* 1960, *15,* 408–411.

Shanas, E. *The health of older people.* Cambridge: Harvard University Press, 1962.

Shanas, E. Social myth as hypothesis: The case of the family relations of old people. *Gerontologist,* 1979a, *19,* 3–9.

Shanas, E. The family as a support system in old age. *Gerontologist,* 1979b, *19,* 169–174.

Shanas, E., & Hauser, P.M. Zero population growth and the family of older people. *Journal of Social Issues,* 1974, *30,* 79–92.

Shanas, E., Townsend, R., Wedderburn, D., Friss, H., Milhoj, P., & Stehouwer, J. *Old people in three industrial societies.* New York: Atherton Press, 1968.

Skolnick, A.S., & Skolnick, J.H. Introduction: Family in transition. In A.S. Skolnick & J.H. Skolnick (Eds.), *Family in transition: Rethinking marriage, sexuality, child rearing and family organization.* Boston: Little Brown, 1977.

Stanford, P. Looking toward the 1981 White House Conference on Aging and beyond: A minority perspective. *Executive summary on the 7th Annual National Institution on Minority Aging.* San Diego: San Diego State University, 1980.

Stuart, M.R., & Snope, F.C. Family structure, family dynamics, and the elderly. In A. Somers & D. Fabian (Eds.), *The geriatric imperative: An introduction to gerontology and clinical geriatrics.* New York: Appleton-Century-Crofts, 1981.

Sussman, M.B. Relationships of adult children with their parents in the United States. In E. Shanas & G. Streib (Eds.), *Social structure and family: Generational relations.* Englewood Cliffs, N.J.: Prentice-Hall, 1965.

Sussman, M.B. The family life of old people. In R.H. Binstock & E. Shanas (Eds.), *Handbook of aging and the social sciences.* New York: Van Nostrand Reinhold, 1976.

Sussman, M.B. *Social and economic supports and family environments for the elderly.* Final report to the Administration on Aging (Grant 90-A-316), January 1979.

Terkelson, K.C. Toward a theory of the family life cycle. In E.A. Carter & M. McGoldrick (Eds.), *The family life cycle.* New York: Gardner Press, 1980.

Townsend, P. *The emergence of the four generation family in industrial society.* Paper presented at 7th International Congress of Gerontology, Vienna, 1966.

Treas, J. Family support systems for the aged: Some social and demographic considerations. *Gerontologist,* 1977, *17,* 486–491.

Treas, J. Socialist organization and economic development in China: Latent consequences for the aged. *Gerontologist,* 1979, *19,* 34–43.

Troll, L.E. The family of later life: A decade review. In C.B. Broderick (Ed.), *A decade of family placed research and action.* Minneapolis: National Council on Family Relations, 1971.

Troll, L.E., & Nowak, C. How old are you? The question of age bias in the counseling of adults. *The Counseling Psychologist,* 1976, *6* (1), 41–44.

Turner, R.H. Role taking: Process vs. conformity. In A. M. Rose (Ed.), *Human behavior and social processes.* Boston: Houghton Mifflin, 1962.

U.S. Department of Commerce, Bureau of the Census. *Historical Statistics of the United States: Colonial times to 1970.* Washington, D.C.: U.S. Government Printing Office, 1975.

U.S. Department of Commerce, Bureau of the Census. *Projections of the population of the United States: 1977-2050* (Current Population Reports Series P-25, No. 704). Washington, D.C.: U.S. Government Printing Office, 1977.

U.S. Department of Health, Education, and Welfare. *Statistical reports on older Americans: Some prospects for the future elderly population* (Department of Health, Education, and Welfare Publication No. (OHDS) 78-20288). Washington, D.C.: U.S. Government Printing Office, 1978.

Valle, R., & Mendoza, L. *The elder Latins.* San Diego: Campanile Press, 1978.

Verwoerdt, A. *Clinical geropsychiatry.* Baltimore: Waverly Press, 1981.

Weeks, J.R., & Cuellar, J.B. The role of the family member in the helping networks of older people. *Gerontologist,* 1981, *21,* 388–394.

Weinberg, J. Of slings and arrows and outrageous fortune. *The American Journal of Psychoanalysis,* 1979, *39,* 195–210.

Weinberg, J. *Mental health: It's importance in total health care.* Talk presented at Eastern Nebraska Office on Aging, Conference on Mental Health and the Elderly: Implications in Continuum of Care, Omaha, September 3-4, 1981.

White, R.W. Motivation considered. *Psychological Review,* 1959, *66,* 297–331.

Williams, R.H. *Perspectives in the field of mental health.* Rockville, Md.: National Institute of Mental Health, 1972.

York, J., & Calsyn, R. Family involvement in nursing homes. *Gerontologist,* 1977, *17,* 500–505.

Chapter 2

An Integrated Model for Family Management

IDENTIFICATION OF DISTRESS ALONG A CONTINUUM OF NEED

Individuals exhibit a wide range of abilities to recognize distress along the life span. Psychological distress in aging can result from perception of normal age-related changes in general health, from signs or symptoms of acute or chronic disease, from perception of change in functional ability, or simply from psychological discomfort. These distresses are individually sensed either directly or indirectly, consciously or unconsciously, symbolically or concretely, vaguely or intensely, quickly or slowly. The individual response to distresses of aging may be subtle or intense, depending on personal and social variables.

Covert and overt symptoms of individual psychological distress can be observed by family, friends, neighbors, or professionals in the environment of the older person. Much distress experienced along the life span is predictable and shared by all; however, responses to distress are extremely varied. Individuals negotiate developmental transitions and physical and psychological changes with varying degrees of adaptive resiliency. Each older person meets the final challenges of life with a different set of life experiences. Each older person construes the continuities and discontinuities of personal and social changes in a different manner; all have shared and varied psychological needs. Physical health is one such need. Good health in old age is possible, but aging clearly increases the frequency, complexity, and chronic nature of disease. In addition, aging increases the severity of acute disease, decreases the adaptive responses of the organism, and decreases the rate of recovery. Disease then becomes a major source of distress and health care a major need for some.

Another emergent concern is the older person's need to sense mastery and control during a period of life characterized by change. Independent functioning is threatened, and the possibility of dependence becomes a source of psychological distress. Cumulative biological, psychological, and social changes, disease, and threats of impaired functioning compromise the older person's thoughts, and another generally distressful continuum of function-dysfunction emerges.

Many of these needs and distresses emerge from gradual change; consequently, continua provide a useful reference. Some of the major continua of needs are as follows: health-disease, independence-dependence, function-dysfunction, social involvement-social isolation, financial security-financial insecurity, self-confidence-lack of confidence. The observation and definition of distress depend upon the interaction of the older person with people in the environment. If the environment is attentive and the aging person is basically trusting, information flows freely and the subtleties of distress are expressed. If the aging person views the environment as hostile or is relatively nonassertive, distress is not expressed by the individual but suffered in silence. Further, if environments lack skilled or attentive people to observe the subtleties, psychological distress remains relatively unnoticed until a crisis point. Families are accessible and available observers in the aging process, and they serve as the first link in definition of expressed and unexpressed distress among members. Families define the *context* of psychological distress, such as onset, duration, and course. Families also reduce the complexity of illness to basic expressive forms separating the good from the bad, the atypical from the predictable, the normal from the nonnormal.

In general, the complexities of distress in the aged have not been well conceptualized by professionals. However, Engel (1960) proposed a unified concept of health and disease that provides a good working frame of reference. Engel states that regardless of the site of the pathology—physiological, anatomical, or biochemical—the *psychological* component initiates the process of defining disease and discomfort. Engel notes further that both health, or the organism's capacity to maintain balance as well as disease, and the organism's failures to grow, develop and maintain balance belong on a continuum. The older individual begins definition of his or her position along this continuum based on the psychological processes of sensation and perception.

These processes begin to define relative degrees of health or disease, the level of function or dysfunction, and the degree of independence or dependence. With this sense of position along a continuum, the older individual may exhibit a variety of adaptive, compensatory, or adjustmental responses. Some individuals may adapt by tolerating distresses without seeking help while others may seek help for mild degrees of distress without attempting less intense resolutions.

The response of others to the perceived distress of the aged is complicated by stereotypical images of the older individual as hypochondriacal, rigid "crocks" or as brave, resourceful stoics, resistant to charity, and "not wanting to bother." The help-seeking behaviors of older people as a group are variously interpreted. Mechanic (1962) proposed a framework for understanding help-seeking behaviors based on how symptoms are perceived. Symptoms are categorized as (1) common, occurring in high frequency in the general population; (2) familiar to the average member of the community; (3) predictable to the outcome of illness; and (4) viewed or perceived from the perspective of the amount of threat and loss likely to result from illness.

Interpretation of this framework in the field of aging points up a number of major concerns regarding the help-seeking behaviors of older persons. Many symptoms of major illnesses occur in higher frequency among older people and consequently could be judged "common" or due to age alone rather than associated with age. Life experiences of the older population very likely familiarized them with a wide range of distress symptoms of their peers, parents, and friends during times when treatments were primitive. Familiarity with the symptoms and fear of the unknown current treatments may adversely affect help seeking. Lastly, the threatening symptom may have little impact on the behavior of older people who are asking themselves, Why survive?

Others have studied help-seeking behaviors from perspectives of socioeconomic class, religion, ethnicity, general stress level, and experience with help seeking. Shanas (1962) points out that the primary reason that older people do not seek medical help remains psychological. All reported evaluations of help-seeking behaviors of older people stress the importance of families in assisting older members to identify distress realistically and to seek appropriate, timely help.

McWhinney (1972) provides additional insight into "patient behaviors" in the help-seeking process. He cites the following considerations: (1) the limit of tolerance for discomfort, pain, or disability; (2) the limit of anxiety concerning the implication of the symptom; and (3) the presentation of a symptom as a problem of living. These relate more closely to psychosocial variables and stresses of the person's life, as Engel (1960) has suggested.

McWhinney's approach has not been applied to the field of aging but it definitely has relevance. Older people tolerate discomforts and pain of illness, ignore the anxiety that symptoms create ("I'll die soon anyway"), and have associated problems in daily functioning because symptoms are far too often viewed as a normal pathway of the aging process.

Elaborate defenses and resistances to initial recognition and identification of distress are varied and unique to the individual and his family. The challenging question for the helping professional is often, Why now? Why has the distress been recognized now? Why does the distressed individual choose to seek help now? What experiences have helped the distressed individual adapt to this point and seek help now?

DEFINITION OF CONTINUUM OF CARE

The concept of *continuum of care* has emerged in response to the evident need for a model that would integrate different levels of distress and provision of services. *Continuum of care* is clearly defined as comprehensive, integrated services including services, treatment, or any type of help with tasks of daily living, provided formally, informally, sporadically, or continually to the functionally impaired elderly. However, practical application of the continuum of care suffers from restrictive interpretation of the concept. The continuum of care is restricted by individual disciplines that see isolated segments of care needs and by service providers who create generic services for individual needs. Program definitions and stated purposes of services (preventive, restorative, rehabilitative, and maintenance) restrict a comprehensive, integrated interpretation. The location of services (home, community, clinic, hospital, or nursing home) restricts the application of the continuum of care across environments (Bernstein & Zander, 1981).

Defining the continuum of care for distressed older persons raises a number of questions. How does the distressed individual define the problem? What one older person defines as a problem is not defined as such by another. What troubles one older person may challenge another. While the continuum of care is a generally accepted concept, various disciplines view the continuum of care differently, usually with their discipline at the center. The continuum of care in one setting may be vaguely defined as a balance of individual needs and supports and in another as a mesh of problems and solutions. Other settings define the continuum of care as a process of diagnosis and treatment of illness and in yet another setting as the optimum fit between a person's needs and his or her natural community support systems.

Individual disciplines providing services along the continuum respond differently because they define only part of the problem. Frequently the acute distress or quickly identified need directs the treatment along the continuum. The urgency of the distress slices the older person out of the continuum of life. The elderly person with chest pain becomes the possible myocardial infarct, and from necessity acute coronary care is set in motion. The person is temporarily removed from the continuum of health-disease at a point where the urgency of the disease directs the continuum of care.

However, at other times, the system of service provision along the continuum unintentionally isolates the distressed from the cause of their distress. The chronic alcoholic gets acute emergency room treatment for alcohol withdrawal seizures only to be returned to the continuum of need in the community and repeat the cycle. Lack of sensitivity to a comprehensive continuum of care by the acute care providers creates longer term inefficiency.

Restrictive definitions of the problem to suit the service providers limit appropriate application of the continuum of care. Nursing homes have been developed as major service providers along the continuum of care and provide a general approach for many specific problems. However, the general nursing home approach has been criticized both popularly and professionally for applying its level of care to people who do not need a high level of care. The continuum of care is restricted to home, hospital, or nursing home. When service providers offer only options of a minimal level of care or a high level of care such as the nursing home, the distressed older person must make a difficult choice. The continuum becomes circumscribed by service models based on efficiency from the providers' point of view. Services are clustered and delivered in mass. General services along the continuum of care isolate the older person from his or her individuality.

Disciplines working within the current continuum of care represent another restrictive influence. Within the arena of service delivery, disciplines tend to function independently. The continuum of care within a medical setting involves a sequence of services: differential diagnosis, provisional diagnosis, treatment prescription, and empirical treatment monitoring. Within a nursing discipline, the continuum of care involves a similar sequencing: nursing assessment, problem lists, care planning, and ongoing nursing support. The continuum of care in social work settings involves intake interviews, case work, and a variety of therapies provided by outreach workers. Psychologists provide personality testing, formulations, and assessments as well as a variety of therapies along the continuum. Educators provide educational assessments and individualized educational plans. In a services for the aged agency, the continuum of care involves screening interviews, referral processes for specific services, and perhaps some advocacy services. Combining these disciplines and service components would represent a working definition of the integrated continuum of care: differential need and differential service provided with flexibility and creativity, giving people what they need when, how, and where they need it.

The related fields of services for the handicapped and mentally retarded offer significant concepts related to the purpose of the continuum of care. Normalization is a keystone in a continuum of treatment environments. *Normalization* is defined as the process of encouraging an individual to function in an environment that approximates normal and enhances the maximum potential of each person served (Wolfensberger, 1972). This idea formed a solid foundation for the deinstitutionalization of the handicapped and mentally retarded and strongly supported the dynamic ideas of continual growth and development. Alternatives along the continuum of care were created for these populations after the theoretical commitment to normalization.

The psychological distress of the aging differs from the distress of the handicapped and mentally retarded. However, the normalization principle is usefully applied. Regardless of an individual's age, there should be energy-driving rehabilitation, restoration of function, compensation, continued skill building and reeducation, approximation of the normal environment, and return to the most therapeutic (least restrictive) care based on improvements and developmental change. The older persons' interest in preserving their normalizing environments is abundantly clear. Antagonistic energy is obvious in the therapeutic nihilism, physician indifference, and the all-or-none kinds of decisions made when defining the continuum of care for older individuals. The normalization principle applied to an aging population would place value on the older person and a positive view of potential regardless of age. Options along the continuum of care would expand.

In addition to disciplines' viewing the continuum of care from varying perspectives, the continuum of care is also popularly but narrowly viewed according to where services are delivered. Specific types of health care and psychological supports can be delivered in the home or community. Public agencies, as well as the private sector, provide in-home supports such as housecleaning, laundry and food preparation services, or home-delivered meals to compensate for milder degrees of functional impairments. Home health agencies provide maintenance and health monitoring functions in home or outpatient clinic settings as well as providing in-home help for maintaining personal hygiene and physical cares. In-home supports and services are available to the older person living alone or with family. Congregate housing with or without congregate meals expands the community-based care options for those unable to maintain a physical environment.

With increasing degrees of functional impairment, the continuum of care options expand to include geriatric daycare centers, day hospitals, senior centers, and structured programs throughout the day to concentrate a variety of outpatient health, psychological, and social services in one easily accessible setting. This continuum of care option allows the older person to function at home with the part-time support of a structured day program. This option also creates day service respite options for the family or primary caretaker. Depending on the degree and nature of the impairment, day services can also be provided through psychiatric day hospitalization or rehabilitation medicine day programs.

Continuum of care options to meet needs of major impairments include acute inpatient hospitalization, cyclic short-term hospitalizations with return to the community, or extended care in a hospital-based nursing home environment. The focus in these more acute settings tends to be restorative. Long-term care or nursing-home care options for major impairments represent the continuum of care options focusing on maintenance and prevention of further decline.

In summary, a practical definition of the continuum of care may include ways to help a sick or disabled older person function in everyday life regardless of living arrangement. Therefore attention must focus on interventions that make a difference in people's ability to work, shop, participate in volunteer activities, cook, clean house, make their beds, choose where they want to live, have fun, and be part of their families—to do all those big and little things that make a satisfying productive life at any age.

EXPANSION OF THE CONTINUUM OF CARE TO INCLUDE THE BIOPSYCHOSOCIAL MODEL

Basic to the provision of care along the continuum is a clear statement of need. Old age in itself is not a need. Needs are determined by the complex interaction of biological, psychological, and social variables. Figure 2–1, the biopsychosocial life-span model, outlines an approach for organizing biopsychosocial variables across time. The left portion of the model outlines the biopsychosocial history of remote past and recent past, leading up to the initial perception of distress. The bridge within the center of the model represents the

Figure 2-1 Biopsychosocial Life-Span Model

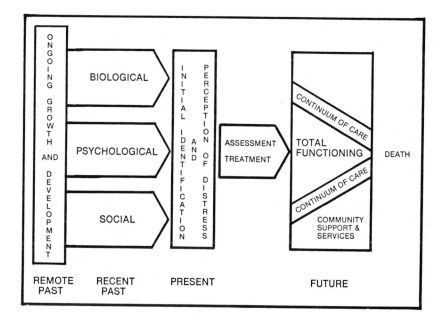

time of initial identification and perception of distress with subsequent bridging to the appropriate services. The right portion of this model represents the change in total functioning of the individual. This level of functioning is variable and support can return the individual to normal functioning. However, graphically, function is viewed as progressive constriction or decline.

These changes in function require compensatory community supports and services defined as the continuum of care. For each current need/medical problem there are biological symptoms, psychological responses, and social reactions. In the case of an older person with evolving pneumonia, the biological symptoms include increased temperature, malaise, headache, and chest pain. The psychological responses may well be anger, frustration, annoyance, or denial. The social responses may well be skipping routine group activities, missing the grandchildren, and becoming housebound.

Each of these biological, psychological, and social responses impacts the current level of care. Current needs must also be understood in terms of recent and remote past dimensions, as outlined graphically. The sum total of the biological, psychological, and social person with an individual history defines the need and subsequently the level of care along the continuum. The older person's perceptions of need also influence the movement along the continuum. Clearly the older person may fear loss of independence or placement outside the home or perhaps tolerate less efficient functioning at an inappropriate level of care rather than risk a move to a different, more restrictive level of care.

The initial psychological distress of changing function, decreasing independence, increasing need, multiple need, and chronic need clearly affects the older person's acceptance of care. Unfortunately, the lack of awareness of the options along the continuum, especially less restrictive options, disrupts the orderly movement into the continuum of care.

The onset, rate, duration, severity, and frequency of distress are important variables in assessing the position along the continuum of care. Also, a clear, comprehensive assessment of biopsychosocial variables is important to complete the understanding of the individual. The older person with a recent hip fracture, good psychological adjustment, and good social direction may need an extended high level of care for the biological problem only. The older person suffering from mild confusion following general surgery may biomedically seem well managed but need in-home support for restoring healthy psychological functions.

The perceived needs of families and their older members interact in complex ways with normative aging processes, individual psychosocial issues, and subsequent social adaptations. The evaluation of need and provision of services must uncover the complexities, relieve the suffering, and facilitate transitions to the appropriate level of care along the continuum.

DEFINITION OF BIOPSYCHOSOCIAL MODEL

The biopsychosocial model provides a means for comprehensive evaluation, assessment of needs, and provision of services along the continuum of care. In order to appreciate the interactive nature of   biopsychosocial variables along this continuum, it is helpful to review the variety of disciplines contributing to the origins of the aging field itself. Professionals interested in aging in the 1980s have searched the repository of knowledge among disciplines to select the information relative to aging, as well as prodding and encouraging interdisciplinary interaction around aging issues. The field of aging has clearly become the property of the creative scientist and the eclectic humanist.

Figure 2-2, of professional disciplines involved in diagnosis and treatment of elderly, reviews the emphasis and overlap of professional disciplines. This graph is by no means complete but it does suggest the complexity of professional perspectives involved in services to the aged.

Figure 2-2 Professional Disciplines Involved in Diagnosis and Treatment of Elderly

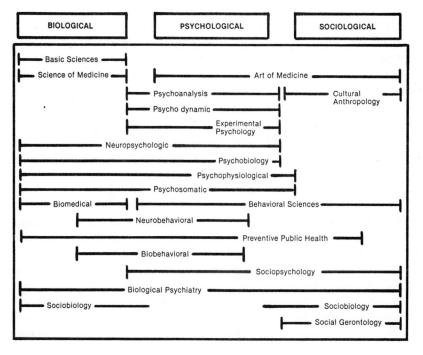

Graphing these disciplines outlines the generally acknowledged biopsychosocial variables. Biological components consist of the biochemistry, physiology, anatomy, genetics, and study of component biological parts such as cells, tissues, organs, and systems leading up to the mind/body dualism. The psychological components include the intrapersonal or intrapsychic "inner life" aspects of both behavioral and adaptive personality styles and responses. This general area defines the makeup of the "person." Social components include interaction of the person with the environment or interpersonal interaction with the family, community, state, country, world, and universe.

A historical review of the advancement of the sciences reveals that the development and elaboration of ideas within each discipline created more highly evolved subspecialty areas. For example, biology and neurology have evolved into neurophysiology. Basic clinical medicine has evolved to include preventive health measures. Psychoanalysis has contributed to experimental psychology, neuropsychology, and the behavioral sciences. Disciplines have expanded, diversified, and realigned around common interests and common problems. However, the field of aging is relatively new to this disciplinary evolution process, and gerontology has been largely a descriptive, isolated science. Contributions to the field of aging have come from disciplines with varying theoretical approaches as well as varying intent, such as education, research, training, and services. Subsequent compartmentalization of these various contributions has been a concern to all involved.

In the field of aging, especially in the 1980s as the field is emerging as broad based and humanistic, the challenge is to *integrate* all information to meet the practical needs of the aging person and to prepare society in general for the aging process. For example, the all too common "tea and toast syndrome" characterized by an older person subsisting on only tea and toast or its equivalent is often viewed independently and in isolation by a variety of disciplines. Nutritional experts approach this syndrome from the standpoint of subsequent calorie restriction, vitamin deficiency, and resulting cellular and system pathology. Clinical medicine views the syndrome as a disease and begins exploring possible causes of appetite suppression, changes in functional capacity, and increased susceptibility to infections. The sociologist approaches this syndrome from a socioeconomic standpoint, concluding that it results from limited income and general disenfranchisement. The psychologist may consider the syndrome as depressive equivalences reflecting poor self-direction, poor self-care and social withdrawal, predisposing low self-esteem, and poor self-concept.

Single-discipline points of view as well as attempts at singular interventions are not appropriate or practical. Moreover, the exclusion of the family from assessment and intervention seems inherently disruptive to the natural setting. Increasing disposable income of the "tea and toast" person through legislation of social programs does not guarantee that the person will readjust psychologically, braving the environment, purchasing more food, and eating it. Provision of more money does not assure that the person will eat nutritionally balanced meals and correct the vitamin deficiency. Psychological readjustment of the person's self-esteem does not necessarily mean that increased food intake will raise albumin levels and restore balance to the biological system. Information regarding the "tea and toast" person from each discipline is clearly needed in order to intervene effectively as well as follow progress of the intervention.

A comprehensive integrated model is urgently needed not only to organize disciplines and guide families but also to organize thoughts, behaviors, and approaches to practical problem solving along the continuum of care for older people. Various disciplines consume resources from within; due to these limitations, comprehensive interdisciplinary approaches may suffer. The lack of resources for integrating interventions and thought in the field of gerontology may be the state of the art or a convenient rationalization. All humanists in the field sense the urgent need for integrated approaches in order to avoid compartmentalization of relevant information, fractionation of interventions, and incomplete interventions. While integrative models demand resources, they more clearly outline responsibilities within disciplines as well as organize information for practical purposes. Clearly, the 1980s technology is creating unlimited options for meeting the challenge of integration.

Kenneth Boulding (1963) has written about the integration process as the "inter-disciplinary movement."

> It may be, however, that what we are witnessing is not so much the unification of knowledge as its restructuring . . . . (f)orced upon us by the very growth of knowledge . . . . There can be little doubt, however, that if the restructuring is under way, it will eventually be recognized officially. Until then, (these structures) will have to live in an underworld . . . of deviant professors, gifted amateurs, and moderate crack pots. (pp. 162–163)

The importance of integrating theory, research, and service approaches is sensed by all in the field of aging. For example, there have been major advances in understanding and documenting the cellular pathology of dementing conditions such as Alzheimer's disease. The isolated discipline of neuropathology has documented the loss of function of a critical mass of nerve cells. The even more isolated discipline of basic research provides an animal model of reactive synaptogenesis (Scheff, 1978) or compensation of nerve cell function by nerve cells that increase function at the synaptic level to compensate for the loss of function of other cells. However, the translation of this information to a memory-impaired, highly anxious victim of the disease demands professional synthesis and creative treatment. The translation of promising futuristic information to a family when the members are already overwhelmed with the victim's loss of basic survival functions seems cruel.

Inherent in the challenge of an integrative model for families of the aged is the responsibility to translate the practical features and promises as well as the current limitations simultaneously. The practical application of information should converge with scientific and research information in order to minimize or alleviate certain psychological distresses.

Development of a model, then, could be approached from two directions: convergence of information from a variety of disciplines to fit the need or divergence of information about the need to fit the available disciplines. The first approach involves integrating ideas, concepts, and information from a variety of disciplines in order to determine what is relevant to the identified need. Development of this model is largely a responsibility of the disciplines involved. The second approach involves elaboration of the practical aspects of the identified need in terms of adaptive capacity or function as observed by the family. Definitions of this integrated model come from the family perspective of need.

The challenge of the first approach, which involves convergence of information from all the relevant and related disciplines involved in the field of aging, would appear overwhelming. Within the last several decades in the discipline of medicine alone, technology and subspecialization have challenged the integrative power of the historically powerful biomedical model. Medicine is increasingly criticized for not treating the whole person. However, medicine is a science based on symptoms and illnesses. Consequently, technology allows measurement of an individual's symptoms of the common cold by a wide variety of sophisticated techniques. Technology creates fashionable subsets of interest, but people still suffer from colds. The clinical application and integration of this vast technology are not, surprisingly, lagging behind. Each general area of biology, psychology, and social/environmental technology feels the effects of tremendous and rapid expansions in the range and scope of their individual subsets of information.

Various disciplines also differ in emphasis on age-related events. Many service-related disciplines continue to operate on a crisis/acute time orientation. Each discipline's contribution to the aging problem solution remains suspect until theories, issues, and practices are viewed against a longitudinal time frame. Integration of the disciplines alone would not result in an integrative posture toward the aging processes. Each discipline would need to consider the time-bound nature of information as well as its dynamic evolving qualities.

The divergent approach to development of a model, while more primitive, appears more relevant. Families continually face practical issues without a large or integrated knowledge base. They begin with a problem, develop possible solutions, and proceed. Consequently, their approach is primarily divergent and potentially incomplete when compared to the biopsychosocial convergent approach. Serial problem solving may be inappropriate for a problem that hasn't been explored in another biological, psychological, or social dimension. The ideal model would include both divergent and convergent thinking for a clearer problem statement and solution.

Biological, psychological, and social variables then reduce and simplify the avenues of scientific approaches and target general points of professional entry into an improved understanding of the human aging process. The particular subset interest, service effort, or primary focus is placed within the biopsycho-social grid of individual aging experiences.

APPLICATION OF AN INTEGRATED BIOPSYCHOSOCIAL MODEL

Application of an integrated model begins with a commitment to education, skill building, and practical experience. Leigh, Feinstein, and Reiser (1980) have applied the biopsychosocial model in educational settings and demon-strated its integrative potential. Continued application in formal educational settings will create a pool of professionals receptive to its application, skilled in its intricacies, and devoted to its results. The concept of teamwork or interdis-ciplinary collaboration is gaining more formal recognition; the details of team approaches and processes are being defined, studied, and refined. The geriatrician/individual aging worker of the future may not face the overwhelm-ing task of integrating diverse sources of information and making judgments in this complex area. The team will define the processes of evaluation, treatment planning, and cooperation in interventions as well as follow up and monitoring with family members as active participants in the entire process.

The burgeoning holistic health movement is encouraging the continued evo-lution of an integrated model. This popularly accepted health movement has been driven largely by younger people, including professionals concerned with maximization of physical fitness, prevention of illness, and control of the risk factors of chronic illnesses. This model appears to have some time restriction; a person's holistic health is sliced from the individual's immediate time rather than his life-span time. However, this holistic model does hold great potential for expansion as older people translate a life history of fractionated care, personal perceptions of health care delivery systems, and current expectations of health care providers into expectancies of holistic health for all generations.

Application of the biopsychosocial model takes many forms and can be used generally or specifically for integration of theory, evaluation of symptoms, or synthesis of case management.

APPLICATION OF THE MODEL FOR CASE MANAGEMENT

The biopsychosocial temporal grid model provides a framework to assess and direct treatment planning of the multidisciplinary team. Use of the model begins with organization of biological, psychological, social variables, and time dimensions on a grid, as illustrated by Figure 2–1, the biopsychosocial life-span model.

Families are often the most valuable resource for past and present information in all three dimensions. Utilization of this biopsychosocial model requires commitment to studying all interaction beyond telephone consultation, quick problem solving, and superficial review. Identification of the purpose of collaboration enhances the treatment function and effectiveness of integrated case management.

The process of assessment and treatment proceeds logically after a preliminary commitment and statement of purpose by the team. Facts are organized in the major components of the grid from various disciplines and sources. Discussion of the potential impact of individual variables on others within the grid is an important aspect and must be done as a multidisciplinary team. Integration of the interactive nature and quality of the entire grid outlines the forces of individual components. The team must identify the primary problematic variables and prioritize them in some fashion.

Advantages and disadvantages of possible solutions to problems must be considered as well as energy expenditures of the proposed solutions. Anticipation of the older person's receptiveness to proposed interventions and the likelihood of cooperation, compliance, and participation in the process are vitally important. Identification of the family's contributions, understanding, resources, and commitment to the proposed evaluation and intervention process is equally important. The team must organize information logically, discuss the interactive nature of variables, and agree on proposed solutions to the problem.

Timelines for the plan and team members responsible for implementing specific parts must be established. Evaluation, monitoring, and problem-solving methods must be incorporated in the initial plan to assure quality, flexibility, and timely adjustment.

Application of this model points up several general cautions. There are limitations in the effectiveness of teamwork in this area of complex distress. The state of the art remains primitive despite widespread commitment to the teamwork process. A professional shortage overloads current workers with more need than available services. Attitudes of older individuals and families toward comprehensive assessment may activate resistance when complete assessments may well involve more time and a series of interviews. A single-discipline approach for a medical problem does not threaten the skeletons that rattle in the family psychosocial closet. The interdisciplinary team must clearly establish definite equality of the disciplines represented and communicate a united front to the older individuals and their families. Obvious conflicts between disciplines of varying educational backgrounds must be neutralized and judgments reserved for the team. This process demands an openness, sensitivity, and honesty of individual disciplines as well as a willingness to admit vulnerability, state-of-the-art limitations of each independent discipline, and shared leadership, given the complexity of the needs.

FAMILY CONTRIBUTIONS AND LIMITATIONS

Families assume a primary responsibility in helping their older members identify distresses from a variety of sources. A number of factors make families best suited for this role. First, families appreciate the continuity of their older members' lives. Older members of families have a biopsychosocial history of function, personality, and health. Beyond these basics, families appreciate the continuity of habits, quirks, preferences, and important daily routines and rituals. This sense of continuity of personality is especially clear in the area of subtle cognitive changes. Families know the history of thinking styles, intellectual interests, and abilities of their older members. Consequently, they may be the first to sense change, question it, and begin interpreting the behavior change.

Families are the silent, unknowing biographers, indirectly recording life events, successful adaptation, and failures of all family members. Their shared experiences provide them the ability to view complementary quirks and habits of older members with a tolerance and humor unmatched by professional outsiders. Their intense motivation, love, and concern fuels their help seeking and advocacy when others are giving up.

With this sense of continuity, families become the most knowledgeable *observers of change*. Complex and subtle changes associated with normal or pathological aging are sensed by observant family members.

Families also sense an older member's *response to change* that may be healthy or unhealthy. They are aware of past response patterns as well as past and present tolerance levels. They know how the older member perceives change and what meaning the change has to the older person. Families sense the mood and humor of the older person. Families know the past, observe the changes, watch the response to change, and interpret its meaning. They provide the context of change and psychological distress.

Families also assume the role of assisting the older members' access to assessment and treatment. Consequently, they are subject to some of the same initial resistances to intervention as the older individuals themselves. They are probably equally influenced by a failure to perceive a continuum of care model, fear displacement, deny problems, and are victims of their own attitudes and bias. Families also are subject to their own adaptive responses of minimization, rationalization, and denial. They may be as limited by their tolerance of pathology and declines in function as the older members. However, the primary limitation of families is their inability to interpret the complete biopsychosocial meaning of change. They must be sensitive to this fact and seek professional help when warning signs of psychological distress appear.

GOALS AND ROLES OF HELPING PROFESSIONALS: SUPPORT, NOT SUPPLANT, FAMILY SYSTEM

Improving the quality of later life in biological, psychological, and social areas must become a unified goal of professionals in the field of aging. Professionals have a responsibility to meet this challenge by overcoming the destructiveness of ageism and realizing how their practices are influenced by age prejudices. The destructiveness of professional turfdom and competition for fame and fortune must be replaced with a humanistic commitment to quality care for older people and their families. The professional community must replace the destructiveness of therapeutic nihilism with timely and quality access to assessment and treatment regardless of age.

In addition, professionals must develop strategies to deal with maintenance-oriented treatment of chronic diseases rather than cure. Professionals must develop strategies to deal with treatment failures. Delivery of services at current state-of-the-art levels must continue while researchers create new models and approaches. When professionals have not participated in relevant training in the field of aging, they must actively seek knowledge through continuing education programs and available community resources.

Professionals must unite, realize their common goals, and learn how to work with older people, their families, and other professionals as a unified multidisciplinary team. This united front demands clarity of multidisciplinary teamwork processes. The roles of professionals working in the field of aging are, of necessity, flexible; often tasks are interchangeable. However, a basic understanding of professional roles is important.

Within the biological professions, physicians have the responsibility for investigating signs and symptoms of illness, separating typical age-related changes from disease, diagnosing disease conditions, and initiating treatment plans. Physicians have the responsibility to family and other members of the team to communicate the meaning of biological change, prognosis, and usual treatment expectations. Reiff (1980) has outlined the medical profession's role in obtaining and maintaining a life medical history.

Nurses also have responsibility for screening and assessing signs and symptoms of disease and referring for more complete evaluations where indicated. In addition, nurses deal with the specifics of how to maintain treatment plans, facilitate compliance, monitor effectiveness, educate the patient, and generally troubleshoot. They assist older individuals with nursing care plans to maintain personal care, diets, and preventive health routines.

Pharmacists have the responsibility for helping the older person monitor medication usage, compliance, effectiveness, and complications. Pharmacists are assuming an increasingly important role in the study of age-related differences in drug absorption, distribution, metabolism, and drug interactions.

Within the psychological professions, psychologists have the responsibility for assessing specifics of personality functioning, cognitive functioning, and behavioral change. Psychologists and psychiatrists share the role of interpreting personality and behavioral change in terms of typical and pathological conditions. They are responsible for guarding, maintaining, and strengthening the personality function of the distressed older person through all types of treatment and services.

Sociologists and social workers have the responsibility for assessing the older person's family, group, and community interactions. Social workers contribute a major treatment component through case work, which involves problem solving, financial management, legal advocacy, and liaison to the larger pool of natural community supports as well as structured resources. Social workers have the major responsibility for meeting family needs.

All members of the biopsychosocial team must appreciate the complexity of psychological distress in aging as well as appreciate the general patterns of aging, distress identification, and help-seeking behaviors. Professionals have a responsibility to respond to concerns expressed by a variety of people who interact with older distressed individuals. The many gatekeepers in the natural environments of older people observe change, perceive distress, and assist the older person seek appropriate and timely help. Professionals need to be sensitive to the varied and occasionally atypical nature of these referral processes.

Professionals must also admit that families' knowledge of older members is superior to theirs in certain areas. As outlined earlier, families know the biopsychosocial history, response, and tolerance patterns and sense the continuity of personality, function, and health of their older members. Families are the best observers of change. While families may lack the ability to articulate this knowledge, professionals have the responsibility to assist them in developing this knowledge base through active interviews and mutual exploration.

Professionals must develop methods, terminology, and means to communicate their provisional as well as definitive diagnosis, prognosis, and expectations to families. Professionals have the responsibility to support the family system, not supplant it. With multidisciplinary professional team support, the family can become the most natural, best-suited, and most knowledgeable case managers for older members. Families naturally are easily accessible and readily available. They assume management responsibilities of sorting out needs and strengths, finding services and supports, and helping their older members through the traffic and complexity of services. With assistance, families can facilitate supports and services as well as evaluate treatment plan effectiveness and advocate for change when necessary. Families can case manage biopsychosocial distresses through the continuum of care with continuity and commitment unequaled by professionals. Their role must not be supplanted.

REFERENCES

Bernstein, S.B., & Zander, K. Continuity of care: A patient-centered model. *General Hospital Psychiatry*, 1981, *3* (1), 59–63.

Boulding, K.E. *The image*. Ann Arbor: University of Michigan Press, 1963 [First published 1956].

Engel, G.L. A unified concept of health and disease. *Perspectives in Biology and Medicine*, Summer 1960, pp. 459–485.

Leigh, H., Feinstein, A., & Reiser, M. The patient evaluation grid: A systematic approach to comprehensive care. *General Hospital Psychiatry*, 1980, *2*, 3–9.

McWhinney, I.R. Beyond diagnosis: An approach to the integration of behavioral science and clinical medicine. *The New England Journal of Medicine*, 1972, *287* (8), 384–387.

Mechanic, D. The concept of illness behavior. *Journal of Chronic Disease*, 1962, *15*, 189–194.

Reiff, T.R. The essentials of a geriatric evaluation. *Geriatrics*, May 1980, 59–68.

Scheff, S.W., Bernardo, S.L., & Cotman, C.W. Decrease in adrenergic axon sprouting in senescent rat. *Science*, 1978, *202*, 775–778.

Shanas, E. *The health of older people*. Cambridge: Harvard University Press, 1962.

Wolfensberger, W. *The principle of normalization in human services*. Toronto: Leonard Crainford, National Institute of Mental Retardation, 1972.

Chapter 3

The Family As a Case Manager and Environmental Counselor in the Continuum of Care

VIEW FROM THE BRIDGE GENERATION

While our society in general is struggling with aging and the aged, the view of the middle or bridge generation is rapidly shifting. We are emerging from a sociohistorical period that encouraged early retirement, bred numerous public support programs, and prescribed a passive role for older nonworkers. Resisting retirement and insisting on continued activity were construed as abnormal and inappropriate (Blau, 1981). The age for social security benefits was lowered to 62 years for women in 1956 and for men in 1961. Compulsory retirement programs drew ideological support from the "disengagement theory," which was popular during the early 1960s (Blau, 1981). The disengagement theory suggested that older persons are naturally susceptible to "an inevitable mutual withdrawal or disengagement" from the mainstream of society (Cummings & Henry, 1961). Popular arguments said that, because disease, decline, and disengagement are inevitable outcomes and characteristics of the aging process, the aged should be made comfortable and excluded, for their own good, from the workplace and sociopolitical participation. Consequently, the older person was systematically disenfranchised and relocated to a marginal position in the American social order.

In the late 1960s, the national view of aging began to change. The disengagement theory became controversial. The Great Society began dealing with these issues by establishing programs and bureaus to operate service programs. In 1965, the Older Americans Act was passed, establishing the Administration on Aging (AoA), mandated "to improve the quality of life of older Americans." In 1974, the National Institute on Aging was created to promote research on the problems associated not only with aging but with physical and mental health throughout the life span. Subsequently, Congress extended the Age Discrimination Act in 1978 to protect classes of workers and job applicants up to the age of 70. Current legislative efforts in the 1980s will undoubtedly encourage individuals to continue to work until 70 or beyond. Many incentives for early retirement have been removed, and numerous public service programs are being dismantled (Peterson, Powell, & Robertson, 1976).

The recent national election embodied several sociopolitical trends illustrating a paradigmatic shift in the government's control and provision of social services that impact care of the elderly. Frankfather, Smith, and Caro (1981) identify the following examples of the shifting view: The government's past and continuing efforts to improve the quality of family life are undesirable; families should not be substantially relieved of traditional caretaking tasks; decision making about care needs and the organization of service delivery should be decentralized; care delivery by professionals is suspect and certainly overextended. While the impact of these ideological changes is not fully understood, it is clear that the sociopolitical definitions of caretaking responsibility for the chronically impaired are in transition. Most elderly are competent during late life; however, at least 20 percent will be severely handicapped in daily functioning and another 30 percent will experience significant limitations in functioning (Frankfather, 1981). Who is to do what for whom? To what extent should society demand filial responsibility for parent care in a culture that has favored serial patterns of responsibility rather than reciprocity? Since each generation has been taking care of the needs of the next upcoming generation, how will the families who are "sandwiched" between generations fulfill new expectations?

In less than 20 years, the view from the bridge has changed radically. Past cultural norms demanded that children honor their filial obligation to their aging parents in a rather undefined manner. Subsequently, the bureaucratization of support services redefined the responsibilities of both generations. Today, after a period of cultural ambiguity, the middle-generation family is to take a more active role in meeting the physical and emotional needs of older members. Similarly, the older person is expected to stay actively involved in the world and off the public dole.

With little experience or knowledge to guide them, families and older members are attempting on a practical level to adjust to the new sociopolitical imperatives. Some families may respond with unnecessary sacrifices in their newly defined caretaking responsibilities. Other families will continue to overestimate the physical health care needs of aging parents and underestimate the older persons' ability to maintain themselves. Still other families will wait too long to seek even partial support for an impaired older person; these families will be forced to choose all-or-none types of care placements. Delays in seeking support or reluctance to seek professional guidance in many cases will result in nearly unbearable demands on the resources of adult children. Feelings of anger, frustration, and despair are disrupting relational patterns, and pseudointimacy between generations clouds the caretaking responsibilities of both generations.

Families usually become most aware of a problem at a time of change, conflict, or crisis such as a serious illness, death of one parent, or other disruption in normal developmental patterns. The family, at these critical points, is assumed to lack specific expertise for dealing with changing events. Often they are encouraged to drop off the problem like a load of dirty laundry to be cleaned, repaired, and pressed by a helping specialist. The specialists, often overwhelmed by the complexities of the problems and beset by their own pessimism, recommend alternative care placements, frequently disregarding the generational interdependencies in the family life cycle. Simple amputation of the older person's problem does not resolve the issues for a family system and the members with interdependent futures.

In order to understand the nature of mutual dependency, the family must be viewed as a system that, along with its elder members, confronts and resolves developmental issues throughout the life cycle. Many of the unmet mental health needs of older persons and their families are associated with unsuccessful assimilation and accommodation of the transitional tasks of later adulthood. When the role or competencies of an older member change, that necessitates change throughout the system. Unsuccessful incorporation of life change events leads to significant disruption in the family cycle. The family is a critical energy source for establishing momentum in negotiating difficult life transitions. This habilitative resource must not be dissipated or lost in the shuffle of out-of-home placement of the problem.

Today's view from the bridge generation is marked by uncertainty and confusion. The bridge generation and the aged themselves lack sociocultural guidelines for growing old. Modern economic currents are undermining historically correct caretaking efforts. Suddenly the Great Society is swept away by inflation and a depressed marketplace. The family's responsibility remains, but who should do what for whom?

There are struggles within families over providing enough financial-emotional support and struggles between families and formal caretaking institutions. The artificial structure of formal caregiving institutions superimposed on the natural system of the family will often have disastrous results. The older person is caught between a desire to live out the natural life span and to hurry death in order to avoid becoming a burden. Some older persons are extremely demanding and seem to live forever, ever increasing their demands on families year by year. Their families are burned out and in this country have little respite for refueling. Other aged appear to content themselves with a few family crumbs on holidays, making minimal demands on the family in hopes of avoiding rejection. Still others—healthy, active aged—resent the demands that adult children may place on them at a time when they prefer to use their limited energy and resources for themselves. Appropriate professional intervention in this hodgepodge of relational attitudes and behaviors is complex. Professionals have their own set of age prejudices and ideas of familial responsibility, which intrude. Everyone has the answer but too many forget the questions.

Examples of family disruption occurring with increasing frequency illustrate the difficulties. The following scenario is repeated over and over with minor substitutions across the country. A middle-aged, childless couple provided a place in their home for the wife's mother during their entire married life. The older woman began to suffer memory losses and confusion, sometimes wandering off day or night, getting lost. Both husband and wife worked; they felt that the cost of full-time supervisory home care would be prohibitive. They decided to place the parent in a nursing home. The wife's sister and brother were furious, insisting that their mother be returned to her home of 18 years. However, both siblings had children approaching college and could not provide additional financial resources nor could they take the mother into their teenager-packed home. Months after the nursing home placement, the families are not speaking to each other. Guilt, blame, shame, and anger prevail (Kalish & Collier, 1981, pp. 206–207).

In another case, Stuart and Snope (1981, p. 146) tell of an elderly couple who lived with their daughter and family in separate quarters of a one-family house. The grandfather developed confusion and disorientation. His behavior was at times bizarre and inappropriate. The daughter and husband argued over the best place for dad. The teen-age son began to stay away from home to avoid the situation. Ultimately, the daughter placed her impaired father in an institution. The mother could not accept out-of-home placement even though she herself couldn't provide the necessary care and supervision. She moved from the house to a high-rise and remained angry and resentful. The daughter and husband eventually divorced and the son left home. The centrifugal forces caused by the grandfather's care needs eventually destroyed the very family who tried to provide the support.

Unfortunately, there are many examples of this type of family disruption and pressure on the "sandwiched" generation and extended families. The lack of information and skill development impeding families stems in part from lack of role clarity and in part from the helping professions' benign reluctance to share the decision-making process with an already burdened family system.

Margaret Blenkner (1965) comments on family role confusion in her description of "filial crisis" and filial maturity. Filial maturity comes from effectively dealing with filial crisis.

> The filial crisis may be conceived to occur in most individuals in their forties and fifties, when the individual's parents can no longer be looked to as a rock of support in times of emotional trouble or

economic stress but may themselves need their offspring's comfort and support. (p. 57)

Successful resolution of the transition to filial maturity involves a mature adult acceptance of a new supportive role—not a role reversal—or child-parent role that accepts and is responsive to the dependencies of aging parents (Blenkner, 1965). The adult child recognizes and accepts the interdependent future of aging parents without invalidating or ignoring the independent past and present.

Typically, as the dependency of the older person increases, the family, dishearteningly, seeks out-of-home institutional care. Institutionalization may appear to be the only viable alternative (Robinson & Thurnher, 1979). Families desperately seek relief from the unrelenting deterioration, grieve for the "living dead," and place the aging parent or relative in a nursing home as a last resort. The absence of services in the community often presses a family beyond tolerance (Brody, Poulshock, & Masciocchi, 1978). Eisdorfer and Keckich (1980) note that

> in England it is possible to hospitalize an older person for two weeks so that the custodial family can take a vacation. In this country, we are horrified at such a waste of money but then proceed to institutionalize the older person for 52 weeks of the year since the family can no longer cope without that vacation. (p. 14)

In addition to emotional costs, the social and economic expenditures of these types of long-term care decisions cost federal, state, and county governments over $14 billion dollars in 1980. The additional cost to individual families for either institutional or in-home community-based care has not been calculated, but fortunately several legislative efforts are directed to relieving the financial burden on families.

As families vary in their resources to provide care, the effects of institutional placement demonstrate similar variability in the impact on the older person and the family system. The effect can be extremely traumatic for all members. Some families, on the other hand, deal effectively with the situation and experience reduced disruption, more frequent and increased quality of contact with older members, and generally improved closeness among family members (York & Calsyn, 1977). It appears that if institutionalization cannot be avoided, involving the whole family, including the person to be placed, when possible in the decision-making process aids in the overall adjustment of the family and older person (Berkman & Rehr, 1975).

Most studies conclude that while families represent a continuum of responsiveness and resources, the presence and willingness of family members to provide care are apparently critical factors in placement decisions. In comparing out-of-home placements with family caregiving, Masciocchi, Poulshock, and Brody (1979) report that two-thirds of the non- and mildly impaired aged in skilled nursing facilities had no families; nearly 80 percent of the severely and totally disabled in the community actually lived with their family. Except for those extremely impaired, it is much more cost-effective to maintain an older person in the community with a coordinated service package provided by both family and formal care agencies than in an institution (Soldo, 1981). Certain caregiving tasks are best done by families but a cluster of care services is best done by formal service networks. The trick is helping families to assess needs and access services.

If families are to be responsible, they must increase their understanding of service options along the various continua of independent versus dependent functioning and the continuum of private versus public reimbursable services. Helping professionals usually discuss continuum of care options in terms of the location of services, from the natural home to an institution. Families often are encouraged to move older members into the "most restrictive" option because "least restrictive" options are not identified or understood. A meaningful continuum of care should reflect not merely the physical location of services but should reflect the person's and family's entitlement to make decisions about medical care. Families are the legitimate gatekeepers of service options because it is in the family that important information about the older person's needs is deposited. Professionals must recognize and accept that the family is the true case manager of care and treatment regardless of the delivery location of services.

The professional's responsibility is not case managing per se but identification of possible therapeutic links between formal and informal caregiving systems. The family milieu provides meaning across the life span and enables acute or chronic impairments to be put in perspective. Meaningful interventions must represent conjoint activity if the well-being of all is to be protected. Families and friends are important in the continuity of care for the impaired elderly and maintenance of the nonimpaired in the community. Informal channels of caregiving exist and are being utilized in some innovative community-based projects, but the family system is the crucial resource.

Families should be helped to understand filial maturity of role changes and to participate in the process if they are to be effective environmental counselors and therapeutic caregivers and to preserve their own boundaries of functioning. Families should be informed as well as instructed so that they may successfully negotiate the developmental challenges of later life including the individual aging of all generations, the decline of members, and eventual death. The helping professions must truly help families in identification, management, acceptance, and incorporation of normal and atypical developmental conflict and change. If the current bridge generation is to be the first to assume a greater share of responsibility for older persons, then they must be included in every step of the diagnostic and treatment processes. Families are more responsive than bureaucracies. However, if families must take more responsibility, similarly they must exert more control. At this time, there are integrated, extended family systems capable of supporting aged dependents, but the professional sharing of decision making is a crucial ancillary service to preserve family functioning. Appropriate service delivery should begin with comprehensive assessment based on actual functioning within natural environments.

FUNCTIONAL ASSESSMENT AND SERVICE NEEDS

Two model community-based assessment programs for alternative services in geriatrics are underway in the United Kingdom and in the United States. These programs are systematically identifying the high-risk, nonclinical aged population for home-delivered care. A family support program in New York is similarly attempting to describe the families' supportive role in delaying out-of-home placement. These programs offer exemplary new approaches to caregiving for the aged and illustrate the emerging contours of home-based family-centered services.

The cross-national geriatric community study (Gurland, Copeland, Sharpe, Kelleher, Kuriansky, & Simon, 1977–78), involving over 850 community residents over the age of 65 from the metropolitan regions of New York and London, is typical of a naturalistic assessment approach to the physical and mental health needs of older persons. This study is significant not only in its scope but also in its shift of focus from hospitalized patients to a community population with much more emphasis on social and environmental factors (physical, interpersonal, familial, and living arrangements). The U.S.-U.K. cross-national project was undertaken in response to the urgent need to improve community services for older persons; the need for refining the differentiation between normal and nonnormal psychosocial changes associated with the aging process; and the need for greater understanding of the etiology of disorders among the aged. It represents a unique effort to examine the use of community resources and services in terms of not only symptoms and need satisfaction of the impaired older person but also the family, household members, or significant others (Gurland et al., 1977–78, p. 3). From these efforts came a semi-structured interview technique called the comprehensive assessment and referral evaluation (CARE). The needs of the older persons are judged on the basis of perceived need by collecting information from the individuals and their families. A follow-up period of one year is included in the study in order to observe the relative impact of mild memory impairments, neuroses, personality disorders, or other minor psychiatric symptoms as those relatively small problems interact and are exacerbated by the stresses of daily living.

The major characteristics of the CARE instrument as noted consist of a series of printed questions or a script that the interviewer reads to the interviewee. The duration of the interview averages 1.5 hours and contains mandatory and contingent questions. A sample question from CARE follows (Gurland, Kuriansky, Sharpe, Simon, Stiller, & Birkett, 1977–78):

> Have you ever felt that you'd rather be dead? (Have you thought of doing anything about it?) If yes: have you felt like that recently? In the last month? Did you actually try anything? When was that? What did you do? What did you plan to do? (p. 12)

The information elicited by the CARE questions or observations of the interviewer is recorded by circling a rating, identifying the relative need for health or social services. The problem is scaled 0 to 9, depending on the intensity, duration, or frequency of the problem. The broad sampling of psychiatric, medical, and social problem areas makes the instrument particularly useful for multidisciplinary community-based teams. Nurses, social workers, paraprofessionals, and physician assistants can be trained to gather reliable clinical information and render a global judgment on the degree of dysfunction, stress, disturbances to others, and dangers to the patient. The global judgments and narrative summaries are easily communicated, if needed, to a treating clinician in a systematic fashion. While the authors acknowledge the need for minor revision in the CARE approach, they have taken a major step in moving the assessment of need from the exit point of an institutionalized setting to the consumer-oriented entry point of community and family.

In summary, CARE is intended to elicit, record, judge, and classify information relevant to the health and social problems of community-based and at-risk elderly populations and their families. It has utility for determining whether an elderly should be referred and to whom. Lastly, CARE, through repeated samples, can be employed in evaluating the effectiveness of the services obtained. This type of comprehensive assessment and evaluation is a particularly useful format for multidisciplinary treatment efforts where systematic communication between team members, elderly, and family is of critical importance.

A second model project of community-based assessment that merits attention is the Older Americans Resources and Service Program (OARS). The OARS project, located at Duke University, is intended to classify the older at-risk population for the purposes of designing care/services systems through the use of a multidimensional functional assessment questionnaire (Duke University Center for the Study of Aging, 1978). The classification schema is a multidimensional approach for assessment of functional levels in physical functioning, psychological functioning, social resources, economic resources, and activities of daily living (Pfeiffer, 1973). Each patient is rated on a six-point scale of impairment for each of the five variables of functioning. A clustering of the cumulative effects of impairments is then determined, based on the widespread clinical evidence that the cumulative effects of specific impairments are more than the sum of individual problems.

In OARS, physical and mental impairments are of primary concern, with either or both causing problems in daily living. Social and economic resources are viewed as modifiers of primary problems. Of course, in reality certain dimensions must be weighed in arriving at a cumulative institutionalization risk score. Pfeiffer (1973) notes that "the presence or absence of a person who can take on major caretaking responsibilities in the household may have *crucial* rather than merely modifying influence on whether institutionalization is required" (p. 14).

Nonetheless, for purposes of general classification, any elderly population, regardless of current living environment, should be divided into classes. From the schema provided by the categories of need, necessary generic services may be identified. A generic service is not tied to a fixed location, mode of delivery, or professional discipline. A generic classification of services allows flexibility in the personnel who will provide the service; e.g., counseling may be provided by a psychiatrist, psychologist, social worker, nurse, pastor, or trainee/volunteer. Moreover, it may be provided in a number of settings, e.g., hospital, nursing home, daycare center, or natural home. The package of generic services identified as required by an aging population contains at least 23 different needs, as indicated in the following list (Pfeiffer, 1973, p. 22):

1. coordination of services
2. counseling-psychotherapy
3. counseling of family members
4. psychotropic drugs
5. medical treatment
6. nursing services
7. physical therapy services
8. recreational services
9. social interaction
10. personal care services
11. food services
12. hotel services
13. legal consultation
14. surrogate services

15. transportation
16. assistance finding paid employment
17. assistance finding unpaid employment
18. vocational rehabilitation services
19. financial assistance
20. "checking" services
21. daycare services
22. "respite" care
23. relocation and placement services

A review of the list of services indicated that, with the exception of hotel service, the services could be provided in a number of settings. The person could go out or the services could be brought into the home. While it may be expedient to put a person with a need for many services in a location offering most of them, it is not absolutely necessary to do so. Pfeiffer (1973) observes that the choice among the options "is essentially a planner's task" (p. 15).

Planning, decision making, and gatekeeping have traditionally been assigned to professional service providers. This arrangement has often left families on the fringe with lots of responsibility, both financial and personal, and little control over the quality of services. Pfeiffer (1973) concludes that the second most important service, next to coordination of multidisciplinary efforts and services, is counseling with family members rather than just serving the older person.

Families are, in fact, the articulator of services whether or not this is acknowledged by professionals; success is dependent upon the way in which the family is included in the assessment-treatment process. However, family-centered care approaches must extend the work of the CARE and OARS projects to include a more directed, integrated treatment orientation. The interactive nature of need, an older person's environmental demands, and the family function as a modifier of impairments is not well understood. Family-centered treatment must look at interventions designed to bring about change but also remain sensitive to the needs of maintenance. The Family Support Project (FSP), which will be described, proposes a maintenance model as a major foundation for building a public policy of care for the elderly through informal family-based support. The Family Support Project, a service and demonstration research project conducted by the Community Service Society of New York (Frankfather, 1981), depicts patterns of stress in family caregiving. The allocation of responsibility and failure of some family members to acknowledge or appreciate each other's contributions at times lead to strained relationships among family members. Strain also results from a lack of agreement on how much or what kind of service to provide. Families reported that they provided support for functionally impaired elderly because of a sense of indebtedness or fear of nursing home placement.

The picture of service style and content emerging from the study revealed that family support is diverse, flexible, generally responsive, and occasionally stressful. The "natural" network of friends and neighbors is more frequently found in professional literature than in reality. Formal services financed through public funds tend to be neither diverse nor flexible (Frankfather, 1981). Those caregiving tasks requiring speed, flexibility, and commitment are apparently best performed by the primary family support groups (Litwak, 1965). The distribution of family activities reported by the FSP and their order of daily frequency is summarized as follows: The number of families reporting that they administer or supervise medication was 41; supervise or assist with personal hygiene, 39; do light housecleaning, 28; visit or make social calls, 28; assist with transfer (moving from bed to chair, etc.) 27; contribute money for expenses, 15; shop for personal items and food, 15; help manage finances, 11; assist in physical exercise, 11; help with laundry, 8; substitute for absent caretaking to assure constant supervision, 8; prepare meals, 4; do heavy housework or repairs, 4; occasionally contribute money for recreation, 3; and assist in transportation, 1.

The 16 categories of support and their reported frequencies illustrate the family's commitment to maintaining the older impaired person in the community; however, assistance is provided according to the caregiver's perception of domestic need. Meeting these needs assumedly prevents or delays nursing home placement. There is little evidence of family-formulated therapeutic plans designed to bring about changes in levels of functioning or improved transactions with family and environment. The patterns of support tend to be reactive rather than proactive as if the families are unaware of the potential of improved functioning. The myth of aging and inevitable decline persists and influences caregiving in subtle, often destructive ways. Families are trying but they lack information and support models for therapeutic or prosthetic interventions. Most importantly, families lack a meaningful problem-solving model for making important decisions about what and where caregiving should be provided.

A decision-making model must begin with definition of the problem. Assessment is the first stage in the development of a treatment plan in or out of the home. Families should be actively involved in each step of assessing, defining, and evaluating treatment of older members. Assessment is a way of systematically gathering information that clarifies and specifies what needs to be done, who should do what, and how to know when it's done. The problems that families bring to the helping professionals are usually diffuse concerns about the older person's level of competence such as loss of memory, disorientation, confusion, and confabulation. The pressing question for families is how these problems in functioning relate to present and future care demands and placement.

In many problems, the disturbance in functioning is greater than could be accounted for by the basic illness or brain impairments. Consequently, the disruption of competence must be influenced by extrinsic factors, events outside the impaired individual. These disabilities have been designated as "excess disability" by Kahn (1966); some may be reversible. Since older persons are more critically affected by and dependent upon their living environments, which includes a family system, it is important to help families look at the older persons' functional capacities within the context of environmental demands and supports. Families tend to focus on the loss of competencies in reference to past levels, which interferes with formulation of the present problems.

The families' lack of techniques for formulating a meaningful problem statement results in an oversimplification or constriction of the available alternatives. An inadequate assessment typically leads to an all-or-none approach to intervention and premature placement of the older person out of the natural home. Persons and environments are always in continuous reciprocal interaction. Competence is a functional relationship between the individual's capacities and environmental demands. Families must be taught to look at and monitor these functional relationships.

Lindsley (1966) makes an important distinction between therapy and prosthetics in caregiving for the elderly, which is germane to the family's decision-making process. Lindsley (1966) defines *therapy* as the traditional approach in which treatment plans are developed to cure the basic cause of illness; e.g., respiratory therapy helps cure pneumonia, psychotherapy helps cure mental illness. He distinguishes therapy from prosthesis, which assumes an unchangeable, nonreversible quality of the disease problem and generates external supports to counteract disability and impairments; e.g., a hearing aid enhances auditory processing by magnifying the sound. Behavioral observation, systematic inquiry, and structured interviews are useful problem-formulation techniques that the family can apply to the interactive nature of competence and care needs in order to differentiate between the need for therapy or prosthesis.

The need for improved assessment approaches led to development of the multilevel assessment instrument (MAI) utilized at the Philadelphia Geriatric Center (Lawton, Moss, Fulcomer, & Kleban, 1982). This instrument identifies seven functional domains as necessary considerations in determining the level of psychological well-being among older persons. These domains are as follows: (1) physical health, (2) cognition, (3) activities of daily living, (4) time use, (5) social interaction, (6) personal adjustment, and (7) perceived environment. Information concerning an individual's achievements in each of these domains is obtained from an informant and from interviewing the older individual. From the preliminary research studies at the Philadelphia center, it is evident that physical health and activities of daily living are robust areas of assessment correlating highly with needed services. The assessment of social interaction and environment and its predictive power is in need of further research (Lawton et al., 1982).

A meaningful assessment approach must be viewed in terms of a continuum of family and individual needs, not a continuum of available formal support service. One must begin with individual and system needs and match need demands to information about the individual and family strengths and deficits within an environmental context. This practice differs significantly from the all too common practice of screening the needy elderly in or out of a variety of care environments.

Traditional assessment approaches too often collect information relative to functional capacity after the elderly have been removed from a natural supportive home environment and family system and without reference to life-span experiences. Moos (1973) observed that "the most important task for the behavioral and social sciences should be the systematic description and classification of environments and their differential costs and benefits to adaptation" (p. 662). Much of the behavioral deviance that families report can be directly understood by limiting environmental factors. The "environmental docility" hypothesis advanced by Lawton and Simon (1968) proposes a similar, if inverse, position, noting that the more competent the organism, the less the proportion of variance in behavior directly attributable to physical conditions, i.e., the environment surrounding the organism. As competence decreases, external environmental factors become more and more important in determining the quality of behavior and feeling. To date, "indexes of incapacity" measures (Shanas et al., 1968) are employed as benchmark measures of home health needs and as planning data for providing support services. These indexes generally review the older person's ability to perform activities of daily living (ADL) and the presence or absence of family, relatives, or friends to assist with ADL if needed.

Lawton's work (1971) improves the indexing system by referring to environmental restraints or facilitators in judging disabilities. The dynamic nature of impairments must be emphasized to an even greater extent in home-based assessment. Traditional approaches to assessing the elderly have generally placed too much emphasis on gross functional changes—i.e., therapy and cure—and too little emphasis on the subtle interactive nature of competency—i.e., prosthetics and maintenance of function.

Home-centered assessment must vigorously borrow from ecological theorists and view the functional capacities of an individual family member in terms of positive and negative deficit transactions within a given environmental context. The interface between individual and environment is at the heart of assess-

Figure 3-1 Diagrammatic Representation of the Behavioral and
Affective Outcomes of Person-Environment Transactions

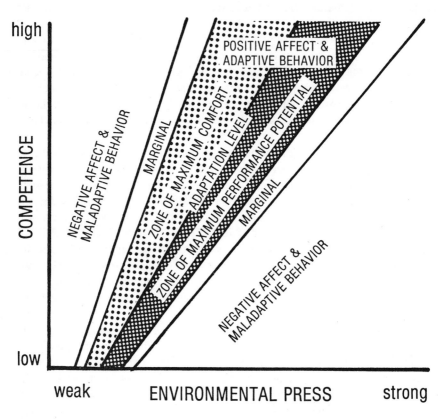

Source: Lawton, M.P. and Nahemow, L., Ecology and the Aging Process. In C.E. Eisdorfer and M.P. Lawton (Eds.), *Psychology of the Aging Process.* Copyright (1973) by the American Psychological Association. Reprinted by permission of the author.

ment as well as treatment. Prosthetic environments can bring about favorable behavioral change in deficient individuals as exemplified by rehabilitative apparatus. Lawton and Nahemow (1973) in their ecological posture suggest that growth and development are more likely to occur when the external demands on the individual are designed so as to be only incrementally greater than the level of demand to which he or she has contemporaneously adapted. Traditional therapeutic approaches tend to exceed incremental ranges whereas prosthetic goals may offer more beneficial matches between the individual response capacity and the environmental demands. The concept of therapeutic environments has not been fully exploited, but they may result in even more permanent changes by defusing pathological forces.

Lawton and Nahemow (1973) offer a graphic description of environmental influences on aging and behavior, as illustrated in Figure 3–1, a "diagramatic representation of the behavioral and affective outcomes of person environment transactions." The model in Figure 3–1 is bipolar in the sense that both high press (stress) and low press (stimulus reduction) are associated with negative outcomes. Changes in competence or in press strength tend to bring about a shift in the level of adaptation; personality, organization, and perception of environmental conditions, of course, mediate the dynamics of changes in adaptation and press levels. This model has some acknowledged limitations and uses several arbitrary concepts such as environmental press, competence, etc. It does, however, suggest the interactive nature of competence and real or perceived environmental demands and the mediation of individual personality styles. As competence decreases, the quality of behavioral outcomes becomes increasingly determined by environmental press, conditions within or external to the individual.

The major assumptions underlining the application of an interactive assessment approach include a belief that the mental health and well-being of an individual should be maximized, regardless of life stage, and that redesigned, less restrictive environments should be considered before moving an individual into more restrictive environments. Treatment goals issuing from these assumptions include interventions aimed at changing the expectations placed on the person, changing the external conditions that delimit the person's functioning, or changing the functional skills of the individual. The problem for professionals as well as families is one of deciding how much support and how much demand to build into a living environment in order that it be optimal for the older person. This problem is further complicated by the diversity of individual living environments and family support system constellations. Assessment must be individualized and guided by flexible principles allowing for personalized treatment for each presenting problem.

Assessment involves the formulation of a problem statement, which includes observations of the individual and environment leading to hypotheses of probable improved functioning. Intervention strategies become test solutions that must be monitored and evaluated. Successes and failures in environmental/individual matches must be reassessed and incorporated into decision-making activities relative to individual competencies and care needs.

Families begin the assessment process by systematically looking at the functional skills of the older person. Functional skills are those attributes that are instrumental in meeting environmental demands. These skill areas may be viewed in terms of the degrees of limitation and compensation for an individual in a given environment. Functional skills may be clustered and directly assessed in the natural home environment or they may be indirectly assessed through interviews with the family or older members. The purpose of assessment is to begin the process of objectifying relevant aspects of the problems and begin the formulation of possible intervention strategies.

For families, the question of competence is the primary problem formulation; secondary levels include questions concerning how the older member should be helped: Is there a best way? a best place to be? Persons and contexts are in a continuous reciprocal interaction. Competence is a dialectic between functional capacity and environmental demands and supports. A functional approach involves looking at the individual and functional skills—skills that are instrumental in adapting to environments. Looking at the environment in terms of characteristics that limit or facilitate accommodation and looking at the individual's transactions with the total environment are most useful. The family is the most important resource in determining competence and offering meaningful descriptions of biopsychosocial functioning.

FUNCTIONAL SKILLS, ENVIRONMENTAL CHARACTERISTICS, AND FAMILY ATTRIBUTES

The aged can be restored to optimal levels of functional capacity through the application of rehabilitative principles (Hunt, 1980). A functional capacities grid based on the indexing approach, therefore, appears to be a meaningful way to handle the initial assessment process in order to plan for restoration and maintenance of function (Marsh, Konar, Langton & LaRue, 1980).

The functional capacities grid depicted in Table 3-1 identifies clusters of individual skills, salient environmental characteristics, and family attributes. Cluster areas include (1) information processing, (2) interpersonal relationships, (3) physical health, (4) self-care, and (5) daily task performance. Under each of these clusters are important skill areas that must be evaluated in terms of their degrees of limitation, which is checked along the scale of asset—no limitation, minor limitation, or major limitation—and checked in terms of the individual or environmental compensation for the limitation.

Information-Processing Skills

Evaluating information processing includes the assessment of the individual's ability and readiness to process either internal or external stimuli. Information-processing skills regulate the intensity of environmental stimuli, the complexity, and the relative proportions of total information that originate from the individual and from the environment. These skills regulate the context of environmental information that is perceived, recognized, or acted upon.

Table 3-1 Functional Capacities Grid

FUNCTIONAL CAPACITIES GRID	ZONE OF ADAPTATION									
	DEGREE OF LIMITATION				COMPENSATION					
FUNCTIONAL SKILLS	Asset	No Limitation	Minor Limitation	Major Limitation	Compensated Fully	Compensated Partially	No Compensation Now	No Possible Compensation		COMMENTS OR COMPENSATION TO BE CONSIDERED
1. INFORMATION PROCESSING										
MEMORY										
ORIENTATION										
DECISION-MAKING SKILLS										
COMMUNICATION SKILLS										
2. INTERPERSONAL RELATIONSHIPS										
MOOD CONTROL										
SOCIAL COMPETENCE										
FAMILY RELATIONS										
COMMUNITY RELATIONS										
3. PHYSICAL HEALTH										
ENERGY RESERVES										
GENERAL										
4. SELF-CARE										
PERSONAL										
DIETARY										
PHYSICAL										
SELF-DIRECTION										
5. DAILY TASK PERFORMANCE										
SPACE MANAGEMENT										
TIME MANAGEMENT										
OBJECT MANIPULATION AND MANAGEMENT										
HOUSEKEEPING										
ECONOMIC RESOURCES										

Source: Degree of limitation and compensation are adapted from S.K. Marsh, V. Konar, M.S. Langton, & A.J. LaRue's The Functional Assessment Profile: A Rehabilitation Model. *Journal of Applied Rehabilitation Counseling,* 1980, *11*(3) 140–144. Reprinted with permission of the Massachusetts Rehabilitation Commission.

Memory. How good is the individual's memory? Are there occasional lapses especially when stressed? Is memory seriously impaired? Is long-term memory good, while the loss of short-term (brief memory like a new telephone number loss) memory is evident? Has the individual family or the environment compensated for memory loss through increased external storage, e.g., lists on the door, telephone reminders, and gentle prompts or cues?

Orientation. Does the individual appear to know where he or she is? What's going on in the world—month, year, upcoming events? What evidence of compensation exists?

Decision-Making and Problem-Solving Skills. Does the individual exhibit the capacity to cope with environmental, interpersonal, vocational, financial, or health-related stresses?

Communication Skills. Can the individual give and receive information effectively?

Interpersonal Relationships

Interpersonal relationships reflect the individual's general capacity to establish and maintain sufficient positive, personal, family, and community relationships.

Mood Control. This involves the appropriateness of affect. Does the individual have awareness and monitoring of moods and emotions? Do the affective responses match the environmental stimuli or is there discontinuity and disruption? Can the affect be engaged through reminiscing?

Social Competence. Mental health is dependent on a positive sense of self, which is formed through and reinforced by social interaction. Self-esteem stems from role adequacy in social positions. Does the person exhibit social competence?

Family Relations. An important developmental change that should be considered is appropriate role dependency, previously described as filial maturity. Is the adult fulfilling a filial role rather than a role-reversed parental role? Does the general tone of family relating appear to be an asset or limitation?

Community Relations. Social space use is determined by the physical distance barrier to mobility and the needed expenditure of energy to access. The critical factors in the ability of older persons to maintain an active social life seems to be proximity to age peers. Segregated housing may have good and bad features. It is important to get some feel for the individual's social support system but it isn't diagnostic. It is not always necessarily the isolate who is placed out of home; quite often it is a highly visible, disruptive person with caring friends and family who is placed in an institution.

Physical Health

Energy Reserves. The adequacy of energy and stamina and the ability to channel energy to activities of daily task performance and leisure plans are considered.

General. Has the person had a recent physical exam? Does he or she have a regular family doctor? Are hearing, eyesight, and teeth adequate or corrected? Can he or she move or sit without feeling dizzy? Can he or she control the passing of urine and bowel movements? What is the general predisposition of the individual to seeking health care?

Self-Care

Review of an individual's capacity to perform tasks in caring for self and the ability to manage one's health and safety needs is important information for decision making. The following areas should be probed.

Personal. Can he or she attend to daily grooming, get on and off the toilet and in and out of the bath, dress and undress?

Dietary. Is he or she maintaining nutritional needs, doing his or her own shopping? On a diet is he or she both knowledgeable and capable of preparing the food?

Physical. Is his or her exercising compatible with capabilities, mobility? Can he or she walk around a room, go up and down stairs, get around in the community?

Self-Direction. A sense of self-direction is important in self-care. Does the individual exhibit goal-directed behavior, perceiving logical steps necessary to reach goals, and follow through on actions?

Daily Task Performance

Does the individual have the capacity to perform tasks and manage the living environment?

Space Management. This is the capacity to move meaningfully from place to place and arrange space to facilitate achievements.

Time Management. Does the person have the capacity to assess needs to manage time efficiently in order to meet those needs?

Object Manipulation. This is the physical capacity to obtain, manage, and utilize tools to achieve an end result.

Housekeeping. Is the person able to organize and implement acts leading to general home maintenance and repairs?

Economic Resources. Given the needs, do the financial resources of the individual or family represent a strength or deficit?

After completing this functional behavioral sampling, the next set of columns is used to indicate whether the person's present use or potential use of alternatives can increase the level of functioning. Individuals who have restored complete functioning in an area are described as compensated fully; those who have made some adjustments in performance of a functional area but who could use additional support are described as compensated partially. The description *No Compensation Now* indicates that the individual has no means of reducing the limitation, but some thought should be given to improving performance. When no method is available to increase the level of functioning, the individual is described as having no possible compensation. Comments are used to note possible courses of action or alternatives.

Having looked at the functional capacity of the individual, it is necessary to look at the environment in an objective manner. Lawton (1980) suggests that an older person is more critically affected by his or her living environment and that, with increasing age, living environments should be increasingly supportive. Competence is defined in reference to functional capacity but it must be also referenced in terms of environmental demand characteristics.

Research studies indicate that certain environmental attributes or characteristics influence the behavior of older persons. These items have been identified by Windley and Scheidt (1980); they are depicted in Table 3-2 and discussed under "Environmental Characteristics."

Sensory Stimulation. To what extent and in what ways can environmental stimulation help compensate for age changes? If, for example, the amount of environmental information received by a person is reduced, redundant cuing could be used to compensate.

Legibility. This relates to the organization and clarity of an environment and the degree to which individuals can identify and structure environmental components in order to form functional relationships. Environments without identifiable components and cohesiveness are likely to increase nonadaptive behavior. The identifiable figure/ground aspects of environments are extremely important to information processing.

Meaning. To what degree does a setting hold meaning for people? Room decor often suggests the relationship between past and present by the types of artifacts, objects, and furnishings in a room.

Sociality. Does the present environmental context encourage or discourage social contact?

Density. To what degree is the space perceived as crowded? Do the living spaces generate age-integrated or age-segregated activities?

Control (Territoriality). Does the individual have ownership of some space in the family milieu? Are spaces designated for certain uses?

Table 3-2 Environmental Characteristics Grid

ZONE OF ACCOMMODATION		COMMENTS OR COMPENSATION TO BE CONSIDERED										
COMPENSATION	No Possible Compensation											
	No Compensation Now											
	Compensated Partially											
	Compensated Fully											
DEGREE OF LIMITATION	Major Limitation											
	Minor Limitation											
	No Limitation											
	Asset											
	ENVIRONMENTAL CHARACTERISTICS*	SENSORY STIMULATION	LEGIBILITY	MEANING	SOCIALITY	DENSITY	CONTROL (Territoriality)	PRIVACY	COMFORT	ACCESSIBILITY	ADAPTABILITY	QUALITY (Aesthetics)

Source: Environmental characteristics are P.G. Windley and R.J. Scheidt's in Person-Environment Dialectics: Implications for Competent Functioning in Old Age. In L.W. Poon (Ed.), *Aging in the 1980's.* Degrees of limitation/compensation are adapted from S.K. Marsh et al., The Functional Assessment Profile: A Rehabilitation Model, *Journal of Applied Rehabilitation Counseling.*

Privacy. To what extent do the features of a setting allow a person to control unwanted stimuli, including people?

Comfort. What environmental conditions contribute to feelings of comfort and ease of task performance, including temperatures, lighting, and other physical aspects of the setting?

Accessibility. The distance to services affects service utilization. Similarly, improperly designed or poorly lit hallways and stairways may be barriers and inhibit normal daily activities.

Adaptability. How easily can a setting be arranged to accommodate new or different patterns of behavior?

Quality. This relates to maintenance and upkeep, size of living space, and aesthetic appeal.

Questioning environmental characteristics generates data relative to important areas of strength, areas of compensation, areas of deficits, and areas of potential change.

Family attributes, the last step in a functional assessment, must also be identified since the family will be the agent of change, as in the primary change agent process. Family assessments should determine how a family, given its particular composition, modes of adaptation, and needs of its members, responds to later-life imperatives. At each stage of a family life cycle, there is a distinctive relational complex for family members with each other. The solution of "problems" of older family members requires, among other things, either a change in behavior or a change in the participants' evaluation of behaviors. In order to plan for change, it is important to obtain a good picture of family attributes, caregivers' experiences, and the promises made, kept, or broken.

Assessing these dimensions among families with aged members poses considerable challenges. However, the clinical literature in aging does suggest some ways to go about this task and how to focus observations and interviews. The key probes in assessing family attributes are listed in Table 3–3, the family attributes assessment. Specific descriptors of family attributes relative to rehabilitative potential are sparse in professional literature. However, a comprehensive overview by Fisher (1976) of assessment criteria relative to family attributes identified five generic dimensions: (1) structural descriptors, (2) controls and sanctions, (3) emotions and needs, (4) cultural aspects, and (5) developmental aspects.

Structural descriptors. These include such things as roles within the family, alliances, interrelational patterns of conflict resolution, perceived boundaries, and views of life, people, and the external world.

Controls and Sanctions. These reflect the rule making and enforcement within the family and the exercise of power in resolution of conflict, including

Table 3–3 Family Attributes Assessment

		ZONE OF ACCOMMODATION									
		DEGREE OF LIMITATION				COMPENSATION					
1. FAMILY STRUCTURAL DESCRIPTORS GENOGRAM	Asset	No Limitation	Minor Limitation	Major Limitation	Compensated Fully	Compensated Partially	No Compensation Now	No Possible Compensation	COMMENTS OR COMPENSATION TO BE CONSIDERED		
WHO											
WHAT											
WHEN											
WHERE											
HOW											
2. CONTROL & SANCTIONS											
FAMILY LIFE REVIEW											
3. EMOTIONS & NEEDS											
ASSISTANCE EXCHANGE											
AFFECTIVE EXCHANGE											
ADAPTIVE COPING SKILLS											
4. CULTURAL ASPECTS											
SYSTEM OF OLD PROMISE											
SOCIAL POSITION											
CULTURAL HERITAGE											
5. DEVELOPMENT ASPECTS											
STAGE APPROPRIATES OF MEMBERS											
STAGE APPROPRIATES OF FAMILY											

Source: Degrees of limitation and compensation are adapted from S.K. Marsh et al. The Functional Assessment Profile: A Rehabilitation Model, *Journal of Applied Rehabilitation Counseling.* Reprinted with permission of the Massachusetts Rehabilitation Commission.

dependence versus independence issues. Although there is some overlap between the first and second categories, there is sufficient separateness to justify splitting the two.

Emotions and Needs. The third area is concerned with probing the emotional climate of the family relative to affective expression, need satisfaction, and dominant affective themes in the family.

Cultural Aspects. These include cultural and subgroup relational preferences, sociocultural views, social status, and any unique environmental stresses from cultural differences.

Developmental Aspects. These involve a determination of individual member's readiness to deal appropriately with age- and stage-related tasks. The life stage of the family unit itself must also be considered.

Information concerning the family structure may be obtained through interviews, self-report at family councils, or use of the "genograms" building technique. Genograms are extremely helpful in determining important characteristics within the family structure. The genogram, by producing a drawing of a "family tree," gathers family history that may be used to project habilitative resources. Guerin and Pendagast (1976) give a good example of the application of the genogram approach. The assessor obtains the names and ages of all members of a family over at least three, perhaps four, generations, asking who entered the family (when and how) and who left it (when and how). The labels that families use for each member reflect expectations as well as experiences. Questions concerning where family members live and who has contact with whom for what reason reveal how families deal with issues of contact and closeness. Caregiving experiences are revealed as families relate major illnesses among members, accidents, or death and similar trauma. Who died? How was it handled? How is the dead person remembered? Who was ill? How did individuals respond? Who took the leadership role for instrumental activities? Who functioned in a supportive role? Who has caregiving experiences?

Factual questions such as dates of birth, marriage, and illness and circumstances of contact or lack of it often stimulate reminiscences about significant moments of promises and ethnic/cultural scripts woven through the fabric of family life. Pursuing family patterns reveals the controls, sanctions, and ways in which members have responded to stresses of life stage transitions and are likely to respond in the present. If the family's adult children have not left home or a grandfather has just retired and moved to Florida or the wife's parents have recently divorced, this is important information in planning change. Stress in families is highest at the transition point from one stage to the next. Symptoms are most likely to appear in a family member when there is an interruption or dislocation in the unfolding family life cycle. A family life review in which members reminisce about significant and trivial memories is important data for predicting how families will deal with the current challenges. Subsequently, therapeutic efforts may be directed toward remobilizing the family life cycle, bringing these combined experiences to bear on current problem resolution.

A family tree may be drawn in order to complement the genogram, including the significant vital statistics of this particular family, and to generate a family chronology. The feelings of family members about the entry and exit points of individuals in that chronological recounting reveal attitudes in providing support for the disabled members (McGoldrick, 1981).

Bengston and Treas (1980) observe that the family solidarity system is composed of the structural relationships reflected in the genogram and the functional aspects such as the quality of interaction and the affects and exchanges of assistance and support. The family's individualistic and cultural norms are illustrated in genogram interviews and family life reviews. Other emotions and needs should be evaluated, such as the amount of time and energy reserves for caregiving that each involved member might have available, the amount of physical and economic resources that might be available, the availability to transport the impaired to services, relative stress-resistiveness coping skills, and the rate of adaptiveness to change. These attributes may be rated positive or negative to give some sense of direction to planning. If, for example, one member has much available time but little surplus income for purchasing services, then a bargain may be struck. Cultural heritage and social position are also generally revealed in genograms or family life reviews. The system of promises or values that operates within a family may be related to cultural patterns or social class. Lastly, developmental aspects must be evaluated. Are family members on schedule in their own life span and is the family on schedule in terms of its life cycle?

Obviously the identification of these family attributes is a non-scientific judgement call, but families themselves are very good evaluators of their own resources. Since families provide the context of meaning for the changes associated with the aging process, family attributes represent an important source of information for treatment planning decisions. The assessment of family attributes is difficult because the more complex the behavioral transaction, the more difficult it is to measure successfully. Nonetheless, we must attempt to measure it. Functional assessment is undertaken not to provide normative or comparative data but to facilitate communication about an individual's ability to meet environmental demands. Changes in functional capacity also may be documented once a true baseline of competency is established. Assessment frees the family from unnecessary dependence on professionals since the effects and outcomes of treatment intervention may be monitored and evaluated by family members themselves.

USE OF ASSESSMENT DATA FOR TREATMENT PLANNING DECISIONS

Now back to the primary questions. Where should the person be served? at home? out of home? If in the home, how? The assessment of functional skills provides us with information concerning the individual capacity to operate and perform tasks most relevant to daily living in the current home environment. The environmental analysis highlights the existing zones of adaptation and zones of accommodation. Should we change the person, change the person's environment, or change both? The family attributes interviews reveal strengths and weaknesses in family resources that may be utilized in conjoint treatment planning.

Once the problem is clearly identified, the next step is to generate alternative solutions. The data from the assessment begin to suggest alternatives. We can create prostheses to ameliorate an "excess disability" or institute therapy to cause favorable change. For example, if daily living and physical health are the main problems, home helpers may be secured. If information processing is the problem, family members may be enlisted to function as prosthetic systems. They can store information, monitor or manipulate mood, or manage behavior. Alternative environments may be explored for partial care or respite. Environmental therapy can be withdrawn or reduced as competence is increased. Decisions about alternatives can become much more systematic, yet diverse and flexible, to meet both individual and family needs.

In many instances, older persons and their families wait too long to apply for more supportive environments, resulting in the "all-or-none," "either-or" phenomenon. Assessment of individual functional skills, characteristics of the environment, and general identification of family resources for responding to the problem results in a refined *problem statement*. The problem is not globally stated as "we must do something about Aunt Mary"; instead, specific limitations and strengths are illuminated. Aunt Mary has degrees of limitations in one or more of the five areas, e.g., information processing, interpersonal relationships, physical health, self-care, and daily task performance. Current configurations in the living environment are increasing or decreasing Mary's ability to adapt or accommodate; e.g., Mary's disorientation may be less if sensory stimulation is increased or decreased or if family interactions are less confrontational and more low-key and reality-oriented. Family transactions could be more supportive, except that Mary has a history of self-centeredness and never helps anybody; the only relative available, a grandniece, has two preschoolers at home and few resources.

Assessment data then are incorporated into a seven-step problem-solving process, e.g., (1) identify the problem, (2) choose a desired outcome, (3) generate several alternative solutions, (4) anticipate the consequences of each solution, (5) choose the best fitting solution, (6) make a plan and implement it, and (7) evaluate the effectiveness of the plan.

The first step for families is to clarify the exact nature of the problem through careful, shared assessment processes. The next step in decision making is to review desired outcomes. In other words, what is an expected and acceptable end-in-view of "doing" something about the problem? Families must at least tentatively decide on outcomes. If out-of-home placement or taking Mary into a family member's home is not acceptable or practical, then the desired outcome is maintaining Mary in her own home or some variation. Families in conjunction with helping professionals should generate several alternatives. This step is like brainstorming. Many alternatives—even outlandish ones—should be identified. It may facilitate decision making at this stage in problem solving to generate short-term (90 days) and long-term alternatives. The fourth step is anticipating the consequences of each proposed problem solution. Families must forecast outcomes but the forecast should be based on quality data, not merely opinion or bias.

Choosing the best fitting solution is another judgment call, but families can increase the quality of judgments by referring to the information gathered in the assessment process. Planning and implementation should be approached systematically and confidently. Evaluation techniques to determine the effectiveness of the plan should be built in, with time limits and criteria. Some forms of record keeping should be decided on and a date of review determined. There is no reason not to anticipate changes in older persons. Families must stay alert to predictable changes as well as environmental influences while keeping the individual's bands of functional competencies as broad as possible. The family is the first link but the role should be more proactive instead of reactive. The family should function as living environment counselors and collaborative case managers instead of arbitrators, reviewing the important aspects jointly as a group that includes older members.

In the decision-making process, families must guard against paternalism, usurping the aged individual's ability to participate in the problem formulation and resolution. Moreover, families must remain aware of their own tendency to overprotect the older person or to tolerate too much disruption and deviancy. Families must be objective if they are to counsel the impaired and nonimpaired elderly. Problem formulation is a way to ensure at least some necessary objectives.

Disability and inability to compensate must be viewed on a continuum from not disabled to slightly disabled to seriously disabled to mentally disabled to severely disabled (Little, 1980). Services are needed in relation to the degrees of disability; however, most services may be delivered either in the home or in institutions. The individual family's ability to be responsive and responsible also exists on a continuum. The helping professional must aid in optimal matching of need and satisfaction; however, the family role in the matching of need/service packages must be recognized and respected. Andrew Hofer's (1981) recent review of eight national family-centered projects indicates that most professionals have not gone far enough in helping families understand the contours of legitimate participation in assessing and treating the psychological distress associated with aging. One hundred thirty-four government-sponsored or -supported programs provide assistance to the aged (Laurie, Walsh, Maddox, & Dellinger, 1978); not one provides clear guidelines on linking informal families' support to formal services.

This section has described community and in-home approaches necessary to family-centered treatment programs. The importance of family participation has been emphasized. The next chapter focuses on specific problems typically reported by families with impaired older members. Subsequently, intervention and home-based treatment strategies are reviewed.

REFERENCES

Bengston, V.L., & Treas, J. The changing family context of mental health and aging. In J.E. Birren & R.B. Sloan (Eds.), *Handbook of mental health and aging*. Englewood Cliffs, N.J.: Prentice-Hall, 1980.

Berkman, B., & Rehr, H. Elderly patients and their families: Factors related to satisfaction with hospital social services. *Gerontologist*, 1975, *15*, 524–528.

Blau, Z.S. *Aging in a changing society*. New York: Franklin Watts, 1981.

Blenkner, M. Social work and family relationships in later life with some thoughts on filial maturity. In E. Shanas & G.F. Streib (Eds.), *Social structure and the family: Generational relations*. Englewood Cliffs, N.J.: Prentice-Hall, 1965.

Brody, S.J., Poulshock, W.S., & Masciocchi, C.F. The family caring unit: A major consideration in the long-term support system. *Gerontologist*, 1978, *18*, 556–561.

Cumming, E., & Henry, W.E. *Growing old: The process of disengagement*. New York: Basic Books, 1961.

Duke University Center for the Study of Aging. *Multi-dimensional functional assessment: The OARS Methodology* (2nd ed.). Durham, N.C.: Author, 1978.

Eisdorfer, C., & Keckich, W. The normal psychopathology of aging. In J.O. Cole & J.E. Barrett (Eds.), *Psychopathology in the aged*. New York: Raven Press, 1980.

Fisher, L. Dimensions of family assessment: A critical review. *Journal of Marriage and Family Counseling*, 1976, *2* (4), 367–382.

Frankfather, D.L., Smith, M.J., & Caro, F.G. *Family care of the elderly*. Lexington, Mass: Lexington Books, 1981.

Guerin, P.J., & Pendagast, E.G. Evaluation of family system and genogram. In P.J. Guerin (Ed.), *Family therapy*. New York: Gardner Press, 1976.

Gurland, B., Copeland, J., Sharpe, L., Kelleher, M., Kuriansky, J., & Simon, R. Assessment of the older person in the community. *International Journal of Aging and Human Development*, 1977–78, *8* (1), 1–8.

Gurland, B., Kuriansky, J., Sharpe, L., Simon, R., Stiller, P., & Birkett, P. The comprehensive assessment and referral evaluation (CARE): Rationale, development and reliability. *International Journal of Aging and Human Development*, 1977–78, *8* (1), 9–42.

Hofer, A. *The emerging role of the family support system for elderly living at home.* Paper presented at the 34th Annual Scientific Meeting of The Gerontological Society of America, Toronto, November 8–12, 1981.

Hunt, T.E. Practical considerations in the rehabilitation of the aged. *Journal of the American Geriatric Society*, 1980, *28* (2), 59–64.

Kahn, R.L. Comments. In M.P. Lawton & F.G. Lawton (Eds.), *Mental impairments in the aged.* Philadelphia: Philadelphia Geriatric Center, 1966.

Kalish, R.A., & Collier, K.W. *Exploring human values.* Monterey: Brooks/Cole Publishing, 1981.

Laurie, W.F., Walsh, T., Maddox, G., & Dellinger, D. Population assessment for program evaluation. In *Assessment and evaluation strategies in aging: People, population and programs.* Proceedings (May 19–21, 1977) of a national conference and related workshops. Durham, N.C.: The Duke University Center for the Study of Aging and Human Development, 1978.

Lawton, M.P. The functional assessment of elderly people. *Journal of the American Geriatrics Society*, 1971, *19*, 465–481.

Lawton, M.P. Psychosocial and environmental approaches to the care of senile dementia patients. In J.O. Cole & J.E. Barrett (Eds.), *Psychopathology in the aged.* New York: Raven Press, 1980.

Lawton, M.P., Moss, M., Fulcomer, M., & Kleban, M.H. A research and service oriented multi-level assessment instrument. *Journal of Gerontology*, 1982, *37* (1), 91–99.

Lawton, M.P., & Nahemow, L. Ecology and the aging process. In C. Eisdorfer & M.P. Lawton (Eds.), *Psychology of the aging process.* Washington, D.C.: American Psychological Association, 1973.

Lawton, M.P., & Simon, B. The ecology of social relationships in housing for the elderly. *Gerontologist*, 1968, *8*, 108–115.

Lindsley, O.R. Geriatric behavioral prosthetics. In R. Kastenbaum (Ed.), *New thoughts on old age.* New York: Springer, 1966.

Little, V.C. Assessing the needs of the elderly: State of the art. *International Journal of Aging and Human Development*, 1980, *11*, 65–76.

Litwak, E. Extended kin relations in an industrial democratic society. In E. Shanas & G. Streib (Eds.), *Social structure and the family: Generational relations.* Englewood Cliffs, N.J.: Prentice-Hall, 1965.

Marsh, S.K., Konar, V., Langton, M., & LaRue, A.J. The functional assessment profile: A rehabilitation model. *Journal of Applied Rehabilitation Counseling*, 1980, *11* (3), 140–144.

Masciocchi, C., Poulshock, W., & Brody, S. *Impairment levels of ill elderly: Institutional and community perspective.* Mimeographed. University of Pennsylvania, 1979.

McGoldrick, M. Problems with family genograms. In A.S. Gruman (Ed.), *Questions and answers in the practice of family therapy.* New York: Brunner/Mazel Publishers, 1981.

Moos, R. Conceptualizations of human environments. *American Psychologist*, 1973, *28*, 652–665.

Peterson, D.A., Powell, C., & Robertson, L. Aging in America: Toward the year 2000. *Gerontologist*, 1976, *16*, 264–270.

Pfeiffer, E. Designing systems of care: The clinical perspective. In E. Pfeiffer (Ed.), *Alternatives to institutional care for older Americans: Practice and planning, A conference report*, Durham, N.C.: Center for the Study of Aging and Human Development. Duke University, 1973.

Poon, L.W. (Ed.). *Aging in the 1980's.* Washington, D.C.: American Psychological Association, 1980.

Robinson, B., & Thurnher, M. Taking care of aged parents: A family cycle transition. *Gerontologist,* 1979, *19,* 586–593.

Shanas, E., Townsend, R., Wedderburn, D., Friss, H., Milhoj, P., & Stehouwer, J. *Old people in three industrial societies.* New York: Atherton Press, 1968.

Soldo, B. When older parents need help. *Changing Times,* November 1981, 80–83.

Stuart, M.R., & Snope, F.C. Family structure, family dynamics, and the elderly. In A. Somers & D. Fabian (Eds.), *The geriatric imperative: An introduction to gerontology and clinical geriatrics.* New York: Appleton-Century-Crofts, 1981.

Windley, P.G., & Scheidt, R.J. Person-environment dialectics: Implications for competent functioning in old age. In L.W. Poon (Ed.), *Aging in the 1980's.* Washington, D.C.: American Psychological Association, 1980.

York, J., & Calsyn, R. Family involvement in nursing homes. *Gerontologist,* 1977, *17,* 500–505.

Chapter 4

Home-Based Habilitation and Maintenance Strategies

FAMILY PROBLEM-SOLVING TECHNIQUES

While each of the professional disciplines involved often views itself as the center of health services delivery and rehabilitation activities, the family remains the important vector of the maintenance and restoration of abilities. Regardless of the designated professional case manager, the family is a social system operating with established protocol behaviors, which support or sabotage habilitative efforts. Families struggling with developmental arrest may be poorly aligned and require special redirection to prevent exacerbation of the older person's impairments. On the other hand, Neugarten (1980) observes that "there are large numbers of families that are going too far in caring for older people, stripping themselves of economic, social and emotional resources to do so" (p. 77). As Neugarten notes, family caregiving patterns, both positive and negative, are "becoming a major source of stress in family life" (p. 77).

The next decades in mental health services will be characterized by a family-oriented, parent-caring managerial balancing act—balancing resources for health and illness; balancing family and individual needs, autonomy, and paternalism; and balancing needs for institutional care against home-delivered habilitation. The mental health and well-being of individuals continue to be related to their families throughout life. Even after years of detachment, families retain the right to evoke mutual responsiveness in times of needs. Kinsmen, as Maddox (1975) asserts, have special, timeless responsibilities to and for each other. Professional caregivers should help families meet these special responsibilities without supplanting the support that families must provide.

This chapter focuses on special habilitative techniques and offers suggestions for both formal and informal caregivers to minimize many predictable distresses associated with the family life cycle and the season of losses. The issue of how much support and how much demand should be built into family interaction patterns for optimum transactions for older persons is complicated by the diversity of needs and the expectation that the aged as a group will become even more diversified in the near future. Chronological age is a poor marker or predictor of needed mental health services or possible family support. Given the variety of needs and the variations between and among families, each of the habilitative approaches discussed in this section is merely a general guideline to be used in individualized problem solving. Each of the strategies must be weighed in terms of individual need, environmental demand, and family resources.

The "terminally" old are treated too often in an aura of specialized diagnostic measurement and evaluation that perhaps inhibits the family's natural rehabilitative efforts. Many mild to moderate impairments can be ameliorated with proper treatment. Frequently, as Butler (1980) testifies, much can be done to reduce the severity of symptoms among even the more seriously involved. Typically, in addition to distress, families report problems in three general areas: memory, behavior, and mood. These problems vary in degree, frequency, intensity, and duration; however, some process-oriented treatment strategies are useful for family-centered intervention approaches. Integrative therapy may be useful in dealing with problems of memory and cognition; behavior management can alleviate many unnecessary stresses; and affect stimulation addresses problems associated with mood states. Lastly, maintenance of balance and boundaries aids in family stress-resistiveness, increases coping skills, and avoids burnout. These four techniques are discussed in the following sections.

INTEGRATIVE THERAPY

Integrative therapy is a tool for reducing memory loss, confusion, and disorientation among the elderly regardless of the severity of impairments. This approach may be applied in formal health care institutions as well as in home-based services. It consists of five process-oriented steps for enhancing cognitive functioning: (1) activation, (2) motivation, (3) habilitation, (4) resonation, and (5) integration. Each step can be implemented by family members individually or conjointly with specific care specialists.

Integrative therapy is based on an information-processing model of brain behavior that escalates the individual's cognitive involvement with present reality through the five processes. Sources of activation or arousal reside typically in past family experiences. The family serves as a primary processing tract throughout development and selected relevant information patterns. Motivation, the second step, attempts to engage the individual and to encourage interest in the selected information. Habilitation refers to specific techniques for repair of skill deficits, which aid in the reconstruction and association of present and past experiences. Current information is then expanded so that it oscillates and reverberates throughout the biological, psychological, and social systems of self-identity. Lastly, the information is therapeutically organized or integrated into the individual's past, present and future experiences. The specific skill deficit training approach is not as important in integrative therapy as the process of guided movement through these five stages of rehabilitation.

Activation

Diller (1976) identified a model of cognitive retraining that includes several interrelated aspects: identification of the defective skill such as visual scanning; selection of a task that adequately reflects the skill in terms of the stimulus properties as well as the response patterns that the task elicits; consideration of the skill and task in terms of daily living needs; the relationship of the desired skill in terms of families of skills; consideration of neurological correlates; and the retraining itself. However, before training can begin, it is necessary to assure optimal arousal of the impaired individual so that the information about the skill is processed or registered. There must be a good match between the skill task demands and the activation of the individual's information-processing system.

Many older persons as well as stroke-impaired patients appear to be under-aroused due to sensory loss, sensory deprivation, medication, or other biological, psychological, or sociological factors. Frequently, brain damage is associated with changes in arousal states since the frontal system of the brain appears to anticipate the information process demands and matches arousal with the task. Dissonance between the arousal level of the autonomic nervous system and the central nervous system results in over- or under-arousal. There is some evidence that in older impaired populations arousal levels are not in harmony, mismatched to the task demands. Consequently, appropriate activation of the older person must be accomplished in initial retraining efforts; alertness must be distinguished from anxiety.

Active involvement with information is a prerequisite for cognitive processing. It is absolutely essential for effective memory behaviors. Stimuli selected to arouse older persons optimally should be chosen on the basis of potential to engage the individual. Highly novel tasks, those with unusual material, or meaningless tasks may not represent good choices. These materials tend to be counterproductive and create even more distance between the individual and the information. Familiar task material and items from the individual's personal and family history may be better choices.

The matching of arousal levels in older persons takes patience. The response time or latency of registration of responses in older and impaired persons is slower. Consequently, the presentation rate should be carefully paced. Multi-sensory approaches, i.e., touch, sight, sound, smell, and movement, may have potential for activation; however, care must be taken not to overarouse, which would also interfere with processing.

Motivation

Motivation is similar to activation but it involves engaging or hooking the individual to relate directly and personally to the information. It conveys a sense of investment, involving the individual's specific interests, aspirations, and goals. Memory and information processing are goal-directed acts; the more meaningful the material to the individual, the more involved or intense will be the interaction. It often is necessary to describe the task or information in terms of its relationship to the individual's goals in order to enhance meaningfulness. Motivation involves not only past experiences but forecasting experiences. Diller's (1976) suggestion of relating skill training to daily living needs is perhaps a critical step in rehabilitation of the aged. It takes a sensitive rehabilitation specialist to broaden the narrow, constricted band of interests found among disabled and older individuals. Direct application of skill training to increase functional capacities, preserve independence, or improve affect is necessary at times.

Habilitation

In order to rehabilitate cognitive losses of an older person, specific deficits in individual functioning must be identified and repaired wherever possible. The professional literature is replete with studies indicating that the performance of older persons in terms of information processing and problem solving is inferior. However, lowered performance appears to be more a function of specific processing strategies rather than due to any major physiological age changes in the neural substrates that support learning activities. One factor contributing to poor performance is the redundancy of many information-seeking behaviors among older persons; i.e., they may ask for the same information over and over. As a consequence they accumulate much irrelevant information and are unable to benefit from their cognitive activity. Excessive negative self-statements also interfere with problem-solving skills. These negative statements are in themselves anxiety provoking, further impeding performance. Before specific habilitation is undertaken, it may be useful to have some understanding of the nature of cognitive functions and the significance of memory losses for the elderly.

Practical Aspects of Memory Loss

Memory is more than simply taking in information, keeping it, and finding it when you need it. Memory allows an individual to accumulate and interpret personal and public experiences. Past and present memories weave the cloth of selfhood and its social connection. When memory is impaired, the inventory or indexing of experience is confused, and the effects ripple throughout the individual's social networks. Memory is dependent upon and reflected in the individual's ability to interpret and adapt to varying social contexts, including the family.

Memory should then be understood in terms of *cognitive* activities rather than in terms of stimuli to be remembered or forgotten. The important focus of memory rehabilitation is on what the individual is doing while preparing to remember. Memory, in this way, is viewed as a symptom or consequence of several cognitive activities engaged in by the individual. Memory is part of a larger brain schema, which is subsumed under *information-processing* skills. Information processing is the way in which an individual achieves, retains, and transforms knowledge. Important to this definition is the concept of organization or how someone goes about reducing the vast amount of stimuli available at any given moment into a manageable, meaningful unit that can be stored and retrieved easily. Moreover, lest we become dependent upon particular stimuli, we must process or organize this information in terms of equivalences so that we may generalize.

Piaget (1954), the developmentalist, noted that memory seemed to be a special case of intelligent activity applied to reconstruction of the past. Materials to be remembered must be incorporated or assimilated into the person's historical sense of his or her own existence or experience. Incorporation also involves motivational decisions about what to disregard and forget selectively. The very sense of self rests heavily upon active memorizing. Consequently, memory impairments may create confusion and confabulation in terms of the self and its relationship to reality.

When faced with a situation in which it is apparent that certain material must be remembered for a future time, like a telephone number, an individual chooses to engage in activities that will maximize the interaction between self and the thing, object, or event to be remembered. For example, the individual may repeat the number over and over or write the number on a piece of paper. These activities maximizing interaction are called *meta memory* or *memory strategies*.

In humans, the unique capacity of the inner or private speech system usually acts as a regulator or selector of these strategies. Memory consists of various cognitive activities and strategies that a person employs to organize information. The individual's relationship to that information is both a cause and effect of memory activities. Remembering is a process of reconstructing past experience, often within the framework provided by the social milieu. Memories without a social grounding tend to fade. Some—not all but some—of the memory loss and confusion exhibited by older patients is related to the drastic changes in their social milieu, which, of course, affects a sense of self and the self's relationship to the world.

The confusion exhibited by a memory-impaired person of selfhood, roles, and relationships is disconcerting to families. The most poignant statement often uttered by family members is, "She didn't know who I was." It is tragic but understandable if one keeps in mind that memory involves the reconstruction of the past, including important past relationships to the self. The research demonstrates that short-term memory is most frequently documented as showing signs of decline in old age (Botwinick, 1981). Long-term memory—the ability to learn new information and development of new skills—persists well into old age (Baltes & Labouvie, 1973; Riegel & Riegel, 1972) and should not be ignored. While some forgetfulness is common in later life, according to Reisberg and Ferris (1982) serious disruption in information processing is not part of normal aging and should be attended to.

Memory Remediation Programs

Programs aimed at remediation of cognitive dysfunctions including memory impairments are not well defined at this time, probably because of the complexity of interplay between social and biological factors. Nonetheless, programs for memory and orientation remediation are often a part of activity programs in health care facilities for older persons. Outcomes of these memory habilitation approaches have been notable in their variability. Reality orientation (Folsom, 1967) is a widely used treatment for disorientation of the elderly and has attracted systematic evaluation of its impact. It is an intensive technique consisting of orienting tasks such as having the patient rehearse the day of the week, the season of the year, scheduled events, and immediate past experiences. Reality orientation has demonstrated more usefulness in organizing staff behavior than in bringing about a significant and lasting change in the patient. It may, in fact, have a negative impact on older impaired patients and should be used selectively (Zepelin, Wolfe, & Kleinplatz, 1981).

Validation therapy (Wetzler & Feil, 1979) has the primary goal of "validation" of the impaired older person's feelings, which then increases the older person's sense of identity, dignity, and self-worth through the therapeutic validating relationship. According to its originators, it has been used successfully to help severely impaired older persons to reconnect with the outer reality of nursing home environments. While validation therapy reports that the older person's sense of self is repaired in terms of the connections between inner and outer realities, its therapeutic goals are somewhat limited, it often excludes the family as an important milieu, and it does not attempt actual reconstruction of cognitive impairments.

The Ebenezer Society (Smith & Gray-Feiss, 1977) also has developed an approach to memory remediation. It uses specific mnemonic techniques such as memory cues, prompts, practice, and motivation to enhance individual memory behavior and increase independent functioning. The memory development program used by the Ebenezer Society is similar to integrative therapy in approach. However, the social context of memory loss and the historical reconstruction of past-present events are incidental rather than intentional in the society's memory development program.

A number of memory activities identified by learning specialists share a facility for increasing interaction between the subject and the object and thus incorporating the material to be remembered. Organization, labeling, materialization, rehearsal, visual imagery, visual and verbal elaboration, self-talk, and stimuli magnification are a few of the natural memory enhancers that can be employed to establish habit bonds or habituation in daily routines. Abundant evidence indicates the importance of organizing activities for memory performance. With increasing age, there is a greater tendency for clustering information. However, many impaired as well as nonimpaired older persons with low verbal ability exhibit an inability to use a "natural" or logical structure in information in order to organize the material for later recall. It may be that life experiences predispose some older people to utilize advanced organizers or structure in the stimuli while others fail even to invent a system. At any rate, material can be grouped or preorganized for the individual, especially along socially familiar lines; improved performance can be monitored for feedback to the individual. Providing external organization for processing while avoiding excessive helplessness and dependency is another rehabilitative challenge.

Labeling is a relatively low-level memory strategy, but it is not a bad place to start. Visually or verbally labeling items to be remembered probably makes the short-term memory trace longer, thereby providing greater opportunity for processing. We cannot learn what we can't discriminate; labeling stimuli may be necessary for appropriate responding. Materialization is a strategy for rendering information into a concrete, material form so that the individual can relate to it. For example, memories may be vague, but looking at pictures and objects from the past renders the memory task more concrete; then a variety of memories can be reactivated.

Rehearsal involves repetition and cumulative practice of the information to be remembered. Programmed learning that is self-paced is a form of rehearsal and is probably very beneficial. The effects of imagery as opposed to verbal context upon recall of information are sometimes difficult to distinguish. Verbal context obviously serves as an aid in inducing visual images. When words are used to evoke very concrete images, recall improves. If the impaired person is unable to construct the sentences, the verbal context of cues that will aid in the construction of an image associating an object should be supplied. Using a place or location to hang a memory has proven particularly beneficial. The longer response or recovery time of older persons, however, needs to be taken into account. The construction of images or association or the visualization of an object and place must necessarily be paced slower to accommodate the individual's cognitive system.

Visual elaboration is a variant of visual imagery in which the subject is taught to make a visual associate or peg on which to hang the material. For example, in a list of 10 pairs of words, visual associations are encouraged. If the pair is tea cup and radio, then the person is asked to visualize drinking tea from a radio. In this system a verbal connection between the nouns seems to facilitate recall. The person must "see" this connection in the "mind's eye." Verbal elaboration is similar except that the images may be less concrete. For example, items to be remembered may be put into a short story.

External storage is a very important technique for extremely impaired persons in transition. In this technique the patient is told to use environment to help structure interaction between self and memorizing. For example, if a person wants to prepare a meal, all items are laid out and grouped according to the sequence in which they will be needed so that nothing is forgotten. Calendars, diaries, date books, bulletin boards, schedules, even family members themselves are good places to store information. Many people who have enjoyed good memories fail to adjust to their own aging process by utilizing external storage devices.

Cognitive behavior management or self-talk is more useful in reducing the task-irrelevant responses of older persons as well as their negative self-statements, which interfere with performance. Self-talk appears to occur naturally in many elderly impaired persons, but this technique stresses how to talk to yourself and get the right answers, answers in terms of providing organization and consistency. Self-talk (Meichenbaum, 1977) is a way of providing external support while avoiding overdependency. We all use it to some extent, particularly when we are confused, frightened, or anxious. It is a way of reducing anxiety and coping via internal speech. The inner statements serve a supportive and guiding function for behavioral responses and direct the self toward the task at hand.

Magnification or intensification of environmental stimuli is a way of arranging information so that it, in fact, has a chance to be processed by the individual. Information to be remembered must be sorted from irrelevant environmental stimuli by separating, as it were, "the figure from the ground." If hearing losses and visual impairments produce a bland, undifferentiated information stream, then it is extremely difficult to focus on relevant informational bits. If the stimuli are separated or intensified, they stand out.

Meaningfulness naturally intensifies stimuli. We pay attention to that which is familiar or to which we ascribe importance. Others in the environment may have to point out or reconstruct the meaningfulness of a person, object, event, or place for the impaired person by relating it to past experiences or current needs. Stimuli may also be physically enlarged or intensified. Several modalities may be used sequentially to process information by telling as well as showing the individual something of importance. Engaging all the senses—hearing, touch, taste, sight, and smell—heightens the stimulus band and may excite the brain to respond more efficiently. Touch, taste, and smell are too often overlooked in communication to impaired elderly.

All of the memory techniques can be explicitly translated into rehabilitation approaches to memory loss and confusion. External memory devices are particularly useful in helping older, moderately impaired persons cope with information retrieval; self-instructional strategies appear to help higher functioning individuals; and externally supplied organizers appear to be best for severe memory impairments. The techniques must obviously be selected on the basis of specific need and current functioning. Diller's (1976) observation that families of skills and neurological correlates must be considered in cognitive retraining programs necessitates a careful analysis of the rehabilitation approach based on a synthesis of available assessment information and the individual's particular needs for daily living.

Resonation

Resonating information involves expanding the event or meaningfulness of a task so that the information reverberates throughout the person's cognitive matrix. The past directedness of older people is well documented in natural and in clinical settings. The function of this past directedness has been defined as adaptive to increase self-esteem, avoid new dimensions, and define a sense of power and personality force (Weinberg, 1974). Reminiscence has been interpreted by Butler (1963) as a healthy process of reviewing life. These gerontologists have set the stage for expansion of the reminiscing process beyond simple memory retrieval. On a more practical note, families involved with older people and the population at large are often in awe of an older person who speaks with clarity about six, seven, or eight decades of experience and memories. This awe is frequently discussed in a simplistic, superficial manner: "He's so alert."

When viewed therapeutically, it is clear that the resonation process of older people involves a continual and evolving definition of the self in present time, definition of self at the time of the retrieved memory, and realization of a sense of change within self and within society. However, the focus on memory research in the field of aging has created general normative patterns that blur the individual and idiosyncratic memory experience. Recent research has focused on subjective and objective qualities of remote memories and points out how the individual's perception of feeling and specifics of remote memories actually change across the life span.

Levels of processing are related to the degree of resonation or reverberation in the cognitive matrix. While the superficial level of information exchange may be defensive in nature, deeper-level processing can help the person reestablish a current definition of self. Resonation then is expansive beyond simple retrieval. It is a recycling of the stimuli of the present time, further identification of stimuli from the environment and from within the individual, resulting in deeper levels of information processing. The process of integrative therapy directs attention to the individualized stimuli, which promotes the resonation and expansion of all possible associations. Families, due to their shared experiences, sense of personal life history, and awareness of life-span interests of the older member, are important adjuncts to resonate the goals process. In other words, families can identify what would encourage a reverberation of memories, enhance retrieval, and aid in redefinition of self. The resonation process then moves like a wave through experiences and cognitive structures.

Affective primers or resonating stimuli are discussed in more detail in subsequent sections; topics of affective import include vocational history, important family experience, achievement, success, and review of earlier peak experience. The goal of the resonation process is to lay the foundation for integrating current information into present time with greater clarity of past, present, and future boundaries, limitations, and potentials. The following example illustrates the ways in which information and memories resonate.

An 83-year-old widow, residing in a nursing home, was plagued with chronic problems of aggressive outbursts involving a physical combativeness, verbal abuse, and at times unintelligible, angry mumblings. These behavioral deficits were overriding a major cognitive impairment; her adaptive maneuvers at times would include feigning sleep, complaining of sickness, and generally withdrawing. When she could be activated, motivated, and taught to attend to conversation, a great deal of her feeling could be consolidated in discussion of previous successful and happy employment as a hostess at an important local restaurant.

In the resonation process, this work experience could be expanded to a discussion of the process of feeding people, the important and well-known features of the menu, the history and experience of the restaurant owner and her family, and other details about that environment. This resonated with the woman's history of experience and definition of self at a happier time and effectively crystalized the personality structure with the cognitive matrix in this process. In other cases, the process of resonation can be accomplished as part of individual psychotherapy with a cognitively intact older person. This process center primarily involves identifying personal events, historically important feelings, and family events; expanding the detail; and realizing greater clarity of personality change over time.

The process of resonation involves initial recall of past experience evoked by some stimuli in the environment or from the inner self. This recall often surfaces in a storybook fashion, which cycles through different levels of processing and expands to include more components of the entire cognitive matrix. Enhancement of this process can be concrete or abstract, depending on the degree of impairment. The cognitively intact are able to provide a history of affective primers including objects, people, places, personal and public events and relationships, vacations, and interests across the life span. These primers are at the base of the cognitive structures and define the personality. Affective primers for the cognitively impaired elderly are discussed in another section. Resonation has significant individual and family value. Shared reminiscing and interfacing on deeper and more meaningful levels aid in locating the current impaired self within a family context. Little can compare to the surprised chuckle or smiling recognition of an older person sharing "I remember" with someone of value.

Integration

The most important and final step is to help the individual organize or integrate current, past, and future information in order to enhance the sense of self and its relationship to the world. This information is thus organized on a heightened level of awareness. The family's and individual's sense of past, present, and future is strengthened. Integration involves putting life events into perspective so that the mind may be more orderly and effective in its approach to current demands.

The integrative aspect of cognitive retraining depends heavily upon communication skills. Families may need practice with active listening techniques or, as Carkhuff (1969) notes, practice with the interchangeable response. The interchangeable response is a conversational reply that includes both the content and the affect of the speaker's statement. It is a rephrasing of what was said, which in essence provides opportunities to validate the speaker's actions. The response is nonjudgmental. Verbal and nonverbal messages are designed to be congruent. The older person's hearing and visual losses may make the interchangeable response and integration of the replies more difficult, but these problems may be circumvented if families and therapists ensure that their responses are brief and clear. Gestures may be used to enhance a message, and voice tone may need to be modulated to compensate for specific hearing losses. Problems with vision may reduce the information usually conveyed by facial expressions, requiring compensation. The personal distance or space between respondents for conversation may have to be adjusted, perhaps making the family member a bit uncomfortable. Shouting may connote aggression and should be avoided. The general slowing of conversation pace must be acknowledged. Response speed does decline, and trying to speed up interaction typically generates anxiety and withdrawal.

The family's involvement at each step of integrative therapy is important. The family may view the cognitive deficits of the impaired person as manipulative and willful, stemming from not trying hard enough, or just plain frightening. Using integrative therapy, the family views the cognitive problems, memory loss, and resulting confusion from a different vantage point and begins to appreciate fully its role as a treatment milieu for cognitive impairments. The family is the primary circle of concern, which has the power to encompass the losses and maintain and restore functioning, aiding all members in meeting developmental challenges.

A FAMILY-BASED APPROACH FOR BEHAVIORAL MANAGEMENT OF FUNCTIONAL DISORDERS AND MORE SERIOUS DISRUPTIONS

Families are increasingly familiar with the challenges of short-term and long-term home care for impaired older members. Older persons frequently exhibit problematic behaviors and attitudes that disrupt the routines and rhythms of family life. Disturbing behaviors are assumed to be an unalterable aspect of growing older. Chronic disruption caused by the older person eventually stresses the family system beyond its accommodation capacity. Efforts to restore equilibrium may lead to premature out-of-home placement. Away from familiar environments, the behavior of the older member further deteriorates. The family's confusion over appropriate locations and duration of treatments is intensified. The displaced older person loses a valuable habilitative setting, and the potential therapeutic benefits of the family milieu are obscured as others usurp the family's roles. Subsequently, weekend and holiday home visits are marked by emotional uncertainties of both families and their older members. Families may wish to reconnect, but they are seldom well guided in their efforts to renew affiliations.

Home-Based Management

This section describes a home-based behavioral management model that professionals may use to help families identify, understand, and modify the behavioral transactions that tend to disrupt family connectedness. Clinical and research observations suggest that behaviors associated with anxiety, depression, and paranoia appear to be particularly disturbing to families and very disruptive of family life. A functional analysis of these behavioral clusters indicates that families could utilize techniques for modifying behaviors as well as encouraging alternative behaviors. Moreover, families can institute preventive planning loops to maintain adaptive behaviors and to circumvent recurrences of problematic transactions. One of the unique aspects of functional behavioral analysis is that problematic behaviors are approached as alterable and improvable until otherwise demonstrated. All behavioral responses, adaptive and nonadaptive, are viewed as complex and reciprocal transactions between the individual and the environment (Rebok & Hoyer, 1977). Sources of variance for disturbing behavioral transactions include the individual's reinforcement history, the history of the current problem behavior, the immediate antecedents and consequences of an act, the reinforcement strength of consequences, forecasting of consequences, and the particular environmental context, including how families think and feel about the particular behavior.

Hoyer (1973) concludes that the way in which the aging process is conceptualized will to a great extent determine the character and utilization of intervention approaches to the pathological aspects of that behavior. If the aging process is viewed as an inevitable decline due to primarily biological facts, then a pessimistic, medically based, custodial model of intervention is used to interpret information to the family and to prescribe treatment solutions. Behaviors such as helplessness, noncompliance, excessive demands for attention, and other dependencies are attributed to natural biological maturation and consequently are not subject to manipulation.

A functional analysis approach, in contrast, conceptualizes all behaviors as learned responses to environmental stimuli. Behaviors operate upon environmental events. Behaviors are strengthened, maintained, or extinguished in association with their consequences. Behavioral deficits are modifiable and nonadaptive behaviors are manageable because of the interactive natures of human response patterns and environmental events. The variance of deviant behavior is not located exclusively within individual biology but in the transactions between an individual and a deficient environment.

The problematic behaviors exhibited by older persons then should be conceptualized as having interactive biological, psychological, and sociological correlates that operate upon specific environments (Hoyer, Mishara, & Reidel, 1975; Labouvie-Vief, Hoyer, Baltes, & Baltes, 1974). Intervention approaches focus upon the behavioral and cognitive transactions of the aging individual with his or her home and family environments. Because the family structure is the arena where transaction occurs, the family milieu is an extremely important treatment consideration in designing primary, secondary, and tertiary levels of interventions.

Understanding Behavioral and Cognitive Transactions

Interpreting problematic behaviors from a biopsychosocial perspective aids families in understanding behavioral occurrences within an ecological or functional context. A number of factors influence the contextual parameters of an action, and families should be made aware of these various factors. For example, families should know that behaviors operate on the environment and are strongly influenced by subsequent consequences or contingencies. The operant approach to behavioral analysis traditionally focuses on the frequencies of behavioral functions within a given context. A great deal of human response is contingent upon reinforcement; intermittent reinforcement schedules are more resistive to change. A behavior that is not reinforced is weakened or extinguished. Conversely, a behavior that is maintained is somehow being reinforced either continuously or intermittently. The exceptions to this statement are those organically driven behaviors that are rarer, even in the aged, than most families suspect.

The behavioral approach deals with observable acts and their operation on environments. Changes in behavior will, in fact, bring about changes in cognition and affect. The family represents a major, and occasionally the only, reinforcement resource in the older person's environment for changing behavior. The rationale for a behavioral approach, as it should be presented to families, is to increase the older individual's functional skills in obtaining positive reinforcements within a given social context. A change in the frequency of a behavior can be brought about through systematic understanding and manipulation of reinforcements available in the environment. Operant methods have demonstrated utility for a wide range of behaviors in the aged, including cognitive behaviors. Cognitive mediation techniques such as self-talk to guide behavioral responses have unexplored but provocative import for managing disruptive behavior in older persons (Hauser, 1981; Meichenbaum, 1974).

In teaching families to use a functional approach to disruption, behaviors are classified as excesses—too much of some behavior—or as deficits—too few operant behaviors for gaining reinforcement or behaviors and cognitions that are inappropriate for the current environmental context. The objectives of intervention are to (1) strengthen and maintain appropriate behaviors and cognitions, (2) weaken or eliminate inappropriate and unacceptable responses, and (3) teach and shape alternative behaviors and cognitions where indicated. The target act must be described in detail, and the immediate situational context in which it occurs must be identified. Observational data relating to the behavior itself, the antecedents or events preceding the behavior, and the consequences or outcomes of the behavior are obtained. Many operant approaches tend to emphasize only three elements: antecedents (A), behaviors (B), and consequences (C) of responding. While many behaviors can be understood with singular reference to the immediate here-and-now, it is more useful to expand the behavioral sample to include information about past and future variables especially when using this approach with families of older persons. Reinforcement histories and forecasts of reinforcements that may or may not be associated with the specific present target behavior should be data gathered for a complete functional analysis. Different family members orient to past, present, and future events in different fashions (Boxer & Cohler, 1980), depending on their position in their own life cycle (Neugarten, 1979).

Kanfer and Saslow (1965) suggest several other areas of observational assessment that must be considered in formulating a functional analysis of behavior. A review of their assessment scheme for these areas includes observation of the following:

- An analysis of the problem situation, which involves specification of the target behavior.
- Identification of antecedents and consequences of the target behavior. Antecedents to behavior are the social and physical settings in which the behavior occurs, the behaviors of others in the setting, and the person's own reported thoughts and feelings within the setting. Consequences are events following the behavior that are reinforcing to the behavior.
- Appraisal of the individual's strengths and weaknesses since a person may have no alternative but to act in a certain way because of behavioral deficits. Identification of strengths and of assets aids in delineating competencies and in producing suggestions for increasing certain needed skill areas.
- Analysis of social relationships, which permits consideration of social networks and identifies whom the behavior is disturbing. In some change plans, the social network itself should be restructured in order to broaden tolerance for "deviant" behavior. The older person's valuing of these social relationships and their meaningfulness is important also in evaluating the problem.
- A motivational analysis, consisting of gathering information relevant to those persons, events, activities, or objects that are reinforcing to the older person. Motivational analysis should focus also on life goal statements as well as on forecasting of expectancies of rewards by the individual.
- Evaluations of the social and physical environment and of the expectations of others, including cultural expectations, are important in shaping behav-

iors. Social roles for older persons, excluding the very rich or very talented, tend to be stereotyped negatively as passive. Consideration of the larger environment is needed to distinguish adaptive from nonadaptive behaviors and aids in the decision whether to change the environment, the person, or both.

- Developmental analysis, involving identification of the historical origins of problem behaviors and of the circumstances surrounding their manifestation.

The Kanfer and Saslow (1965) model provides an extremely useful guide to observational assessment and data gathering. A model of observation for understanding behavioral transactions, depicted in Figure 4–1, represents an expansion of Kanfer and Saslow's descriptions in order to include past histories and future forecasts of target actions. The model is presented to families, accompanied by an explanation of how behavior is influenced by past, present, and future contexts.

Developmental History

A brief developmental history should be obtained in order to establish some idea of the older person's past behavior as well as to identify relevant current environmental changes. Some problem behaviors may have been adaptive earlier in life for specific environments and are no longer adaptive because the environmental demands have changed (Zarit, 1980). The current problem may have a rich and elaborate reinforcement history involving the entire life span of the individual. A developmental history may also reveal whether the problem behavior originated earlier in life and if so, what treatment was effective then in changing the behavior.

Current History

The current history of the problem in conjunction with its developmental history identifies sudden shifts or changes in the environment that may have affected the availability of reinforcers. Losses in the environment that typically accompany aging, such as sensory losses, memory losses, social losses, loss of status, and loss of independence, all can result in relatively sudden changes in behavioral response patterns. Fear of additional loss expressed through forecasting and simultaneous removal of historically available reinforcers may in fact account for much of the current maladaptive behavior. Current history also aids in differential diagnosis of chronic from acute biopsychosocial events.

Antecedents-Behavior-Consequences

The problem behavior (B) must be described with particular reference to its frequency (e.g., five times a day), its intensity (mild, moderate, severe), and

Figure 4-1 Understanding Behavioral Transactions

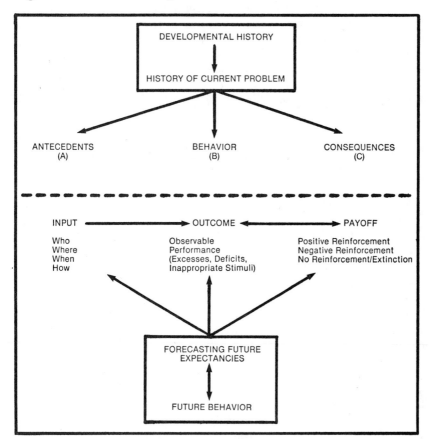

Reprinted with permission of *Clinical Gerontologist,* 1982.

its duration (minutes, hours, days). The input characteristics or antecedents (A) are clarified by observing who is involved in the transaction, when it most frequently occurs, and how the behavior is exhibited. The payoff or reinforcing consequences (C) of the behavior may be judged positive, negative, or neutral. The observational questions are, What happens after the behavior? and How does the person exhibiting the behavior appear to feel about the consequences? At this point, a decision must be reached by the family regarding whether the problem behavior is modifiable or is sufficiently disturbing to justify the focused energy needed to change the response patterns.

Generally, families have difficulty in pinpointing specific behaviors and instead report global behavioral clusters. Teaching families to observe behavior accurately is sometimes the greatest obstacle to applying functional analysis. A few practice sessions with videotapes of routine behavioral transactions are usually sufficient to sharpen the observational skills of families. Once the family has become familiar with targeting problem behavior, the members are encouraged to formulate a more refined judgment of the behavior by using a simple decision tree. Since most maladaptive behaviors are really normal responses that occur too often, too little, or at inappropriate times, family members are instructed to think about behaviors in terms of excesses, deficits, or inappropriateness. For example, a family member should consider, Is a behavior disturbing because of deficiencies or lack of responses given the environment? Is the behavioral response beyond the stimuli of the environment, as with paranoid ideation? Problems involving excess behaviors are usually easier for families to identify than cases of deficits or of inappropriate stimuli.

Once the behavior has been specified, the family must attend to the antecedents and consequences. Simple recording devices or baseline methods are used as aids to observation; family members should exchange information in order to refine their sampling techniques. Interrater reliability of an observational sample can be obtained by having two family members count the same behaviors within a period and compare their counts for agreement. If two or more family members describe the antecedents, behaviors, and consequences, their descriptions should agree at least 80 to 90 percent of the time.

Forecasting and Future Behaviors

Traditionally an operant analysis approach to behavior seldom emphasized forecasting or developmental histories in determining a change plan. It has been argued that change in the immediate here-and-now behavior will obviously change future behaviors and that history cannot be changed. In a functional analysis approach, more consideration is given to developmental histories and forecasting. The older person's forecast of reinforcements, or the lack of reinforcements, is important to understanding many disturbing behaviors associated with anxiety, depression, and paranoia.

Anxiety

Anxiety, for example, may be formulated as an excess of negative forecasting based in free-floating, fearful anticipation of loss, fear of disease and illness, or fear of failure to adapt and be acceptable within the social context. Fear of additional loss in conjunction with too few or inadequate coping skills to deal with loss impacts current behavior in a number of anxiety-producing ways. Many times in an effort to protect and care for older family members, we overprotect. Overprotection communicates our own fear that the older person lacks the competence and control to adapt and adjust to present demands as well as to those of the future. Additionally, the older person may lack a clearly defined current or future positive role in the family system, which further erodes confidence. The family in its caring may in fact inadvertently arrange the older person's environment so that there are reduced opportunities to exhibit competence or control. In an effort to minimize stress, the family may remove the very challenge that would enhance the older person's sense of competence.

Many combative and noncompliant behaviors exhibited by older persons center on issues of rigidity, control, and fear of loss of competence. If anxious behavior can be identified as excessive negative anticipation in conjunction with deficits in coping skills for dealing with more loss, then the family may routinely handle management of anxious behavior in a number of ways. The family can structure the immediate environment in ways that increase the older person's sense of control over the environment. The family should allow the older member the security of daily living routines without encouraging preoccupation with routine. Older persons should be encouraged to participate in long- and short-term decisions relating to family life. The content of anxious behavior should be identified and labeled instead of generally dismissed with the proverbial "don't worry." Opportunities for expression of competency should be reinforced and expanded whenever possible.

A family's general plan for response to anxious behavior may include increasing the older person's sense of control over the environment, decreasing fearful behavior by identification and discussion, and encouraging alternative behavior that might result in more positive forecasting. Moreover, the family might selectively rearrange antecedents so that stress is reduced but not eliminated and encourage the older person to encounter the situation. Behaviors can also be redirected so that different consequences can occur; alternative behaviors, such as relaxation training, may be taught. In order to reduce anxious behavior, the family should seek to promote and maintain the emergence of an independent personality who is involved actively in the world.

Depression

Depression and depressive symptoms such as insomnia, despair, lethargy, anorexia, loss of interest, and numerous somatic complaints represent the most prevalent psychiatric disorders in old age. While substantial literature links depression to changes in brain structure and function, most instances of depression in older persons are in fact independent of organic impairments. Depression is also linked to social and psychosocial changes such as role restriction, grief and mourning, and "learned helplessness." Depression in older persons is obviously complex and involves both organic and nonorganic etiology. Minimally, depression does involve construing experiences negatively, viewing one-self negatively, and viewing the future negatively. Regardless of origin, depression involves a deficit of responses that might secure positive consequences and an excess of negative statements about the self in relation to past, present, and future events. Since depressed people do not exhibit many reinforceable behaviors, the lack of positive reinforcement then contributes to feelings of sadness, helplessness, and worthlessness, all of which further decrease the output of acceptable behaviors. In a sense, adaptive behaviors have been extinguished.

Seligman (1975) characterizes depression as "learned helplessness," which relates to a sense of powerlessness to affect the environment or secure reinforcements. Feelings of powerlessness are increased when the reinforcements are not contingent upon behavior. Families often reward or reinforce the older member for dependency and for expressions of helplessness. In a sense, the older person is rewarded intermittently with attention for not acting. Behaviors that are learned on a schedule of variable or intermittent reinforcement are more difficult to extinguish. Inadvertently, the behavior is in fact shaped and strengthened because only the more extreme manifestations of the behavior are attended to. A family management approach to depression consists of restructuring the environment (antecedents) as well as defining the reinforcements (consequences) so that rewards for behaviors may once again be contingent. Negative self-statements are consistently ignored and positive self-statements are expanded through immediate and consistent reinforcing attention.

In managing depressive illnesses, there is a need to encourage the person to "decenter" the preoccupation with negative forecasting. Inactivity and isolation appear to exacerbate depression as well as to reduce the opportunities for positive reinforcement. The family may need to reduce expectations initially so that even minimal responses are reinforced. Arranging the environment in order to encourage active involvement is effective in reducing depression. The older person also can be given new skills in managing and controlling reinforcement contingencies through self-management of behavior. For example, the older person can be encouraged to substitute self-awareness statements for self-critical ones, thereby using proportionately more positive than negative self-statements. Bayne (1971) suggests that it is not only by controlling and modifying the environments of others that we can help the elderly but also by teaching them to modify and create their own environments and contingencies. Thus older persons can become active participants in change plans as well as maintenance plans for reinforceable behavior.

Paranoia

Paranoid states occur less frequently than depressive illnesses in the elderly, but their impact is often greater. Reports of delusions concerning intruders, thefts, plots, and voices, suspiciousness, and distrust are likely to be very disturbing to family members, particularly since the family itself is often identified as part of the problem. Families tend to react, in fact overreact, quickly and negatively to paranoid statements. Whereas depression is more a matter of deficit behavior, paranoia reflects current and forecast behavioral excesses that apparently are not under control of any mutually agreed upon stimuli in the environment.

Paranoid behaviors appear to be associated with at least two, and probably more, etiological tracks: deprivation or omissions, and guilt or commissions. Sensory, social, and environmental deprivations often lead to a situation in which the distinction between the world out there (reality) and the inner world of self becomes blurred. If there is a low rate of sensory and social input due either to physical and environmental conditions or to the person's own difficulty in assimilating input, as in the case of certain forms of memory impairment, then disorientation and hallucination might occur. Hallucinations might even be maintained for the stimulation that they provide. Many older persons live under conditions of sensory deprivation, isolation, memory loss, and confusion, experiencing only fragments of reality. Paranoid ideation may be an attempt to put the pieces into some meaningful, consistent, and connected, albeit unrealistic, world.

Paranoia also appears to be associated with guilt feelings about a variety of issues including unresolved sexual needs; survival when others, such as a child or spouse, die; and an almost catastrophic reaction to one's own progressive losses. Paranoia in the aged is not fully understood. Nonetheless, treatment must be initiated and should be directed toward the emission of alternative behaviors that are most appropriate to the environmental context. The family should withdraw reinforcing attention to paranoid statements and develop alternative reactions that are incompatible with, but not confrontational to, paranoid beliefs. The family might respond briefly in a concerned manner to the delusional statement rather than argue about whether something occurred and should move quickly to reinforce other statements. Families should be prepared to introduce and discuss other topics and issues of interest so that the elderly may move beyond delusional statements. Families should attempt to eliminate any payoffs for paranoid acts and to reconnect the older person's attention to other environmental contingencies. Increased stimulation and increased social connections to the ongoing flow of the real world aid in decreasing paranoid delusions.

Paranoia ideation may be manifested in a variety of behaviors. Paranoia is complex and, like depression, may represent a continuation of a longer-term psychiatric problem originated at an early stage in life and requiring ongoing professional help. However, only a minority of persons exhibit the more extreme and bizarre symptoms characteristic of paranoia schizophrenia, which requires intensive professional help. Many paranoid delusions of older people may require only moderate levels of professional intervention, preferably within the family milieu; they are often transitory in nature.

Procedures for Home-Based Management

Of the procedures discussed, then, the operant method emphasizes that the frequency of behavior is associated with the amount and type of reinforcement or punishment resultant from these behaviors. The functional approach directs attention to the environmental context. The behavioral transaction approach expands these concepts to include forecasting. In applying these concepts to home-based management of problem behaviors of older persons, the family is instructed to (1) specify the behavior precisely; (2) take a "before measure" of the behavior, usually a frequency measure; (3) identify the A-B-C pattern; (4) develop a change plan that takes into account developmental history; current history; strengths and weaknesses; the motivation of the person; social, cultural, and physical aspects of the environment; and the forecasting of the individual; (5) initiate a plan for behavior that targets singular or combination change decisions to increase a behavior, decrease a behavior, extinguish a behavior, or maintain a behavior; (6) manipulate the consequences and the antecedents or provide contingencies for alternative behavior once the direction of behavioral change has been decided; (7) continue to measure the behavior; (8) determine a reasonable trial period; (9) communicate changes periodically; and (10) regroup in order to make adjustments in a systematic fashion as indicated when a change plan is not working.

In setting up a workable change plan, families are instructed to target only one behavior at a time. All steps of the plan should be agreed upon by all members who will be involved, including the person whose behavior is being changed. The disturbing behavior is likely to escalate initially. The person may try harder for the habitual reinforcement as rewards are withdrawn. Families are encouraged to stick with the plan long enough to give it a fair trial. Most families report that they have tried such and such in the past and it didn't work. The emphasis on objective recording of behavior frequencies and on advance agreement of all members on a single behavior change, in writing, usually circumvents this resistance. When a plan is not succeeding, the family might need help with problem solving for the intended changes.

There are a number of common disruptions to behavioral functioning, particularly among organically impaired populations and chronically mentally ill populations. These disruptions affect behavior management techniques in major ways and are consequently discussed at this time. It is frequently difficult in some cases even to begin modification of behavioral dysfunction due to the extensive variety of target behaviors, their diffuse nature, and the great range of underlying causes for behavior disruption. Cognitive impairments that affect temporal and spatial disorganization as well as memory functioning may make it difficult to sequence antecedent behavior and consequences. Emotional instabilities similarly present problems in that the ability to modulate and generalize affect appropriately in response to a behavioral sequence is impaired.

These problems could also be organized in terms of a continuum of more primitive and disorganized to more abstract and psychologically driven. These are discussed in a hierarchy ranging from the most primitive concrete behaviors to the more abstract. The more abstract psychological issues, of course, are influenced by more intense emotional charge, resulting in discontinuous behavioral sequences, manipulation of people within the system, and motivation composed of intention, future orientation, and reasonable expectation for reward.

Intervention in these problem areas is complicated by the intense interrelationship of the biopsychosocial variables. Nonetheless, the following primer of interventions may be helpful in handling even the most challenging problem.

Problem Behaviors

The behavioral sequence A-B-C may be totally unrelated, resulting in random responses as illustrated by Figure 4–2. It may be impossible to relate a behavior to either antecedents or consequences due to its random nature. It is possible that unrecognized or unobserved antecedents or consequences are acting within the environments or within the individual. It is important to stay aware of the random nature of behavior; avoid labeling the behavior as purposeful, intentional, or motivated; and redirect the individual's acts where possible. Figure 4–2 depicts possible sources of behavioral variances in cases where antecedents and consequences are not properly related.

Dealing with behavioral dysfunction as a result of impaired reality is complicated by the fact that behavior sequencing is often stimulated by an old antecedent in time, place, or person. Mistaking a person—perhaps a stranger, children, relatives, or friends—may set in motion behavior unrelated to the current reality. Other behaviors can be explained in terms of disorientation to place, such as the appearance of the home environment suggesting another, earlier environment. Behavior in the current reality is based on misperceived stimuli, precipitating seemingly unrelated responses. Intervention for this group of disruptions involves (1) teaching orientation to time, place, and person; (2) reviewing the old antecedents of current behavior or the old antecedents offered and resonating with past experience, connecting them to present reality; and (3) using the technique more as a coping mechanism than intervention by recogniz-

Figure 4–2 Behavior Modification Model for Specific Problem
Behaviors

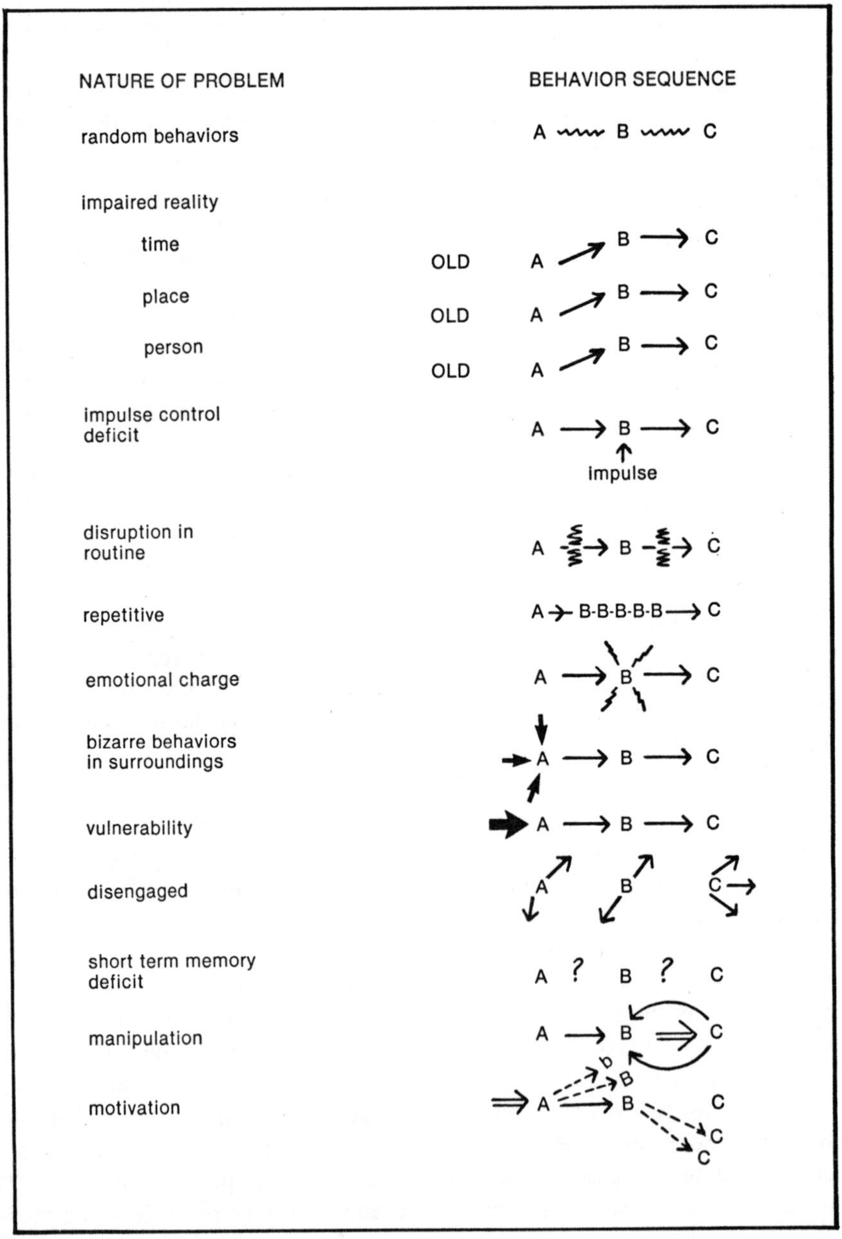

ing the need for intervention and avoiding discouragement with minimal successes.

Behavioral disruptions subsumed under problems of impulse control occur when an inner impulse drives the behavioral sequencing irrespective of the antecedents or consequences. Intervention focuses on teaching the individual how to identify inner meaning of the impulse. This may not be possible if the person is experiencing serious cognitive impairments. It may be necessary simply to control this type of impulse-driven behavior externally.

Disruption in routine often results in behavior-sequencing problems and acceleration of problem behaviors, especially in the obsessive-compulsive personality types. It should be noted that obsessive-compulsive ritualized behaviors may represent an adaptive response in cognitively impaired persons to order their illogical world. Consequently, disruptions in routine are disrupting to the entire personality structure. Interventions involve reassurance, approximation of the usual routine, and teaching.

At other times behavioral dysfunction is a result of a repetition of behavior when stereotypic antecedents do not lead to desired consequences. This behavior may reflect major cognitive impairment or it could be an obsessive-compulsive adaptation. It may also represent the responses of a higher functioning person who is simply bored. Interventions involve evaluating the exact nature and desired consequences of behavioral repetition, confronting and shaping it in its most appropriate fashion.

Behavior with an emotional charge is very common in impaired elderly when an antecedent stimulates an overreaction. Interventions involve exploring the interactive nature of biopsychosocial variables, empathizing, reducing tension, and humoring when appropriate. Bizarre or aberrant acts often disrupt responses in higher functioning people because the predictable environment has been changed. Intervention should be to reassure, support, and segregate the bizarre acts. Intervention involves reintegration of the person into a stable environment as quickly as possible.

Vulnerability becomes an issue in behavior management on several levels, particularly when the older person is obviously susceptible and vulnerable to direction by a variety of powerful outside sources. Intervention involves being aware of one's ability to influence vulnerable older persons and being aware of how they may be influenced by other people within the environment.

The issue of disengagement involves a disruption in the behavioral sequencing in that the antecedents may not be connected to the behavior or to the consequences due to the disruption in the person's engagement in sequencing, in receiving, etc. Interventions involve reengaging and redirecting. In cases of short-term memory impairment, the person cannot remember the antecedent. Consequently, behaviors operating in a very immediate or urgent fashion are either driven by direct and immediate stimuli or not directed at all. The clear

A-B-C sequencing is lost, and the person gets caught up in current behavior problems. Interventions involve teaching the sequencing, offering others in the environment as external memory stores; and developing cues in the environment to aid control.

Family members may feel manipulated by the impaired older person. The antecedent-behavior-and-consequence sequence seems to be clear with reinforcement of getting one's own way. Interventions include a clear evaluation of the pattern, changing the consequences by ignoring or withdrawing, while keeping in mind the manipulative person's ability to substitute other behaviors and escalate the demands. It is important to be aware of one's own feeling and avoid overreaction. A common misunderstanding is to attribute manipulative intent to only the impaired person when actually in managing behavior we become manipulators for our own reasons.

Summary and Implication of Home-Based Management

Adaptive and maladaptive behavior is learned. Behavior operates either directly or through cognitive mediation, e.g., forecasting upon the environment. Behavior is maintained, strengthened, or weakened by consequences that it elicits or the anticipation of consequences. Changes in behavior often bring about changes in thoughts and feelings but only through cognitive cooperation. The goal of a family-based management plan is to increase the older person's skill in obtaining positive reinforcement for successful adaptation to daily living within a family system. Families should be aided in identification of problem behaviors and given the information and skills that will enable them to manage behaviors more appropriately, on either a long-term or short-term basis.

The key to teaching families behavioral management techniques is behavioral rehearsal with a therapist. The "dry run" of management is an extension of the behavioral assessment process. Liberman (1981) suggests that families formulate a sense that stimulates the main features of the problem behavior and practice their strategies. Modeling the appropriate manner of intervention and shaping in small steps successful participation may be helpful for families who lack skills in management. Management techniques in general range from actual behavioral modification of responses—i.e., providing complete extrinsic environmental control of behavior—to less directive techniques that involve the target person more in the decisions about behavior such as writing behavioral change contracts or psychotherapy. The amount of extrinsic versus intrinsic control needed must be decided, case by case, given the behavior of the person. Generally, independence should be preserved, and the family should use only as much externally directed control over behavior as the problem warrants.

A home-based management approach may delay out-of-home placement of the older person, thereby assuring the family's availability as a habilitative resource for the predictable mental health needs of an older person, or it may facilitate reentry of an impaired member. In general, it would appear that the family milieu should be used increasingly as a normalizing vehicle for delivery of many preventive and educational aspects of mental health services as well as for conjoint treatment of certain aspects of mental illness. Consequently, it is necessary for professional health care providers to broaden their clinical treatment knowledge to include naturalistic settings such as the home environment and to expand their data bases to encompass successful resolution of problems in daily living in the normal home environment. The new professional must be able to translate knowledge into the vernacular of family routines and articulate the treatment demands of individual family members with the needs of the total family system.

AFFECTIVE STIMULATION

Aging is associated with complex physiological and psychological changes that apparently disrupt socioemotional interest and investment in activities of daily living. While there has been little research directly exploring mood, emotionality, and emotional behavior in adult development, Schultz (1982) believes that it is possible to predict intraindividual developmental changes by extrapolation from known biological and social-psychological changes. Since individual affect, mood, or emotional states influence a person's social cognitions, memory efficiency, and general tendency to pay attention to available environmental information, emotionality is an important but relatively unexplored area in aged behavior.

Buss (1973) differentiates emotion, mood, and affect on the basis of intensity or underlying level of arousal. For example, a highly aroused behavior such as rage could be considered an emotion while less aroused states such as dissatisfaction are more characteristic of moods or affects. Brady (1970) suggests another useful distinction between moods and emotions based on the locality of the behavioral environment; moods are most often located within the individual. Schultz (1982) adds still another possible descriptor of emotions and moods in terms of duration of the state from temporary to enduring. Emotions may be relatively short-lived whereas moods may persist over time. Valence, or the attachment of negative, neutral, or positive value, does not differentiate well between emotions and moods but would apparently affect the individual's level of arousal.

Krathwohl, Bloom, and Masia (1956) separate affective processes from other cognitive activities and place affective responses in the following hierarchy: (1) receiving—the willingness to attend to certain stimuli; (2) responding—active involvement with the stimuli; (3) valuing—appreciating or expressing the worth of a person, object, or event; (4) organizing—ordering values into a system; and (5) generalizing—integrating values into a work view or philosophy. It is evident that these affective processes are considered along with cognitive operations in the application of integrative therapy discussed in an earlier section; e.g., activate—increasing appropriate attending; motivate—increasing participation; habilitate—increasing opportunities for investment in persons, objects, and events; resonate—organizing and associating information with past valued persons, objects, and events; and integrate—generalizing from past experiences and incorporating present experiences within the matrix of personality. It is also evident that disruptions in investments and problems with modulation of mood and emotional control may be directly addressed within the context of the family milieu or within other care environments. Mood and affect may or may not be influencing emotionality, depending on the environmental context.

The affective impairments of the elderly are seldom directly probed by the helping professionals. Schultz (1982) notes that data describing affect and mood are less available than data on emotional states. Cameron's (1975) study of mood is perhaps the most comprehensive investigation. Mood states of 6,452 persons aged 4 years to 99 years were assessed; no significant age differences were noted in the frequency of reported happy, sad, and neutral moods. Lawson (1978) reviewed research on the subjective well-being of older persons and found well-being to correlate strongly with physical health, followed by social economic factors and social relations including marital status, housing, and daily mobility, or availability of transportation. No differences in subjective well-being were reported as a function of age alone. Therefore, aside from biophysical changes, serious disruptions in emotionality, mood, and affect are not a part of the normal aging process.

The process of identification of affective investments and feeling states/responses has also been shrouded in the mystique of psychoanalysis. Popularization of feeling expression seems to be associated more closely to a younger population—getting in touch "with feelings," or the "gut level." The image of the older person's affective life is restricted and limited. Culturally, we may be shutting out older persons' feeling expression, ignoring it, or not recognizing it because it is more subtle or highly intellectualized but not verbalized in the current vernacular. The elderly do sense a lack of congruence between their current self and the current social context. Dissonance may stem from the elderly's slower registration of environmental stimuli, from less efficient auditory and visual scanning of environmental stimuli, or from social disconnectedness due to losses in role, goal, and norms to guide interactions.

The elderly experience restricted areas of affective expression; families can play an important part in expansion of affect. Regardless of the degree of cognitive impairment, the affect domain may be impacted if approached systematically. The authors have successfully used affective stimulation with

Exhibit 4–1 Affective Primers

What _____ have stimulated
strong feelings in you as:

	Young Adult	Mid Adult	Older Adult
1. Objects/Things			
2. People			

3. Places/Environments
  a. familiar/known
  b. unfamiliar/unknown			

4. Personal, local or national			
5. What other relationships, pet or acquaintances			
6. What work or chore			
7. What non-work or vacation activity			

chronically impaired patients and less impaired community-based patients. The affect abilities training program described here offers guidelines for the seriously impaired, institutionalized elderly. Affective primers may be used with mildly disrupted elderly to begin a systematic exploration of life span, emotional investments, and changes.

Affective Primers

Emotional redefinition and expansion of current affect may be facilitated through the use of affective primers. Erikson (1964) states that "living together means that the individual life stages are interliving" (p. 14). Families have interdependent futures as well as interdependent pasts. Several techniques may be used to gain information about past experiences that may be used to "prime" current affective expression in exchanges between the family and older members. In order to know what is truly important now in a person's life, it is important to know what was important. A list of affective primers that can be used to stimulate shared exploration of valued experiences is provided in Exhibit 4-1.

Table 4-1 Sample Life Chart

Biopsychosocial Event	Year
Birth	1917
Foot Injury	1921
Kindergarten	1922
Broken Arm/Baptized in Episcopal Church	1925
Confirmed/Entered Jr. High/Began Band	1928
Entered High School/Band/Chorus/Speech	1931
Injury to Hip-Lifetime Handicap/State Legion Citizen Contest (first notice of "you are very smart")/First Date	1934
High School Graduation/Named Regent's Scholar/ Entered University of Nebraska	1935
Attended University of Nebraska - No Money -Drought - Depression	1936
First Teaching Job ($630 per month)	1937
Teaching & Summer in College	1938
Teaching & Summer in College	1939
Return to College/Rejected by Draft - Physical	1940
Graduated from College	1941
Married	1948
Daughter Born.	1952
Vice Principal	1959
Passed Over for Promotion	1960
Stomach Problems/Active in Community Group	1961
Took New Job	1962
Granddaughter Born	1970
New Job Responsibilities	1972
Daughter Divorced/Daughter and Granddaughter Moved Away	1975
Passed over for Promotion/Raise	1977
Divorced - Wife Retired	1979
Remarried	1980
Sister's 50th Wedding Anniversary	1981
Decision to Continue Current Employment	1982

Another technique for gathering information relative to affective primers that families may use is a modification of the life chart (Meyer, 1948). Individuals are asked to fill in important biological, psychological, and social life events. The sample life chart, Table 4–1, was completed by a distressed 64-year-old male facing retirement. A review of life change information with his family stimulated discussion concerning his sense of despair over a level of accomplishment. His achievements did not match his family's promise for him. Preretirement counseling centered on possible second-career options and the development of leisure interests to provide alternate routes of achievement. It is also therapeutic to review life charts that have been completed by several family members in order to gain some sense of individual world views, attitudes, interests, motivational patterns, and possible points of arrested development in the family life cycle as well as future expectations.

In some cases, it is helpful to use family photograph albums as affective primers. Entin (1981) reports that the use of family photographs aids in identification of important family events in the family life cycle such as births, weddings, holidays, reunions, and even deaths. The minislice of the family's past helps to illuminate generational themes and provides "landmarks for a history of continuity and change." The stimulation from the photographs also provides an excellent jumping off point for therapeutic life review and reintegration of present relationships within their sociohistorical family context.

Weinberg (1974) wrote poignantly about past and present communication between generations in a discussion entitled "What Do I Say to Mother When I Have Nothing to Say?" He observed that adult children must learn to listen creatively, hearing not only the manifest but latent symbolic content. The implicit poetry of life review holds the keys to current reengagement to impaired and nonimpaired elderly. Weinberg (1974) concludes that adult children must learn as well to hear the silence—that which is left unsaid—and determine what must be said, shared, or redefined.

Older persons express a need for improved communication with their adult children or other family members. The Ebenezer Center for Aging and Human Development developed an exercise to stimulate affective transactions between adult children and their aging parents that might facilitate understanding and relating between generations (Carroll & Costello, 1979). The exercise, "How Well Do You Know Your Aging Parent," is a list to be answered by adult children. "How Well Do Your Adult Children Know You" contains similar questions to be completed by the parent. The two sets of answers are then compared for areas of congruence and areas of divergence.

Dissonance in communication can usually be traced to differences in what an individual believes to be true generational differences in values. There may be substantial differences between generations in terms of value judgment about behavior. Schaie (1981) relates value differences to four stages of development:

acquisition, achievement, responsibility, and reintegration. During the acquisition stage of childhood through young adulthood, instrumental-material values appear to dominate. The young adult in the achievement stage strives to achieve by integrating role independence with the assumption of responsibilities. There is a decline in instrumental-material values as well as an increase in personal growth values. The responsible stage is characterized by a decrease in personal growth interest and an increase in interpersonal-expressive values. The last stage of reintegration occurring in late life is marked by selective attention to egocentric meaningfulness and a renewed increase in instrumental-material values, with hedonistic values particularly manifest in older males.

Understanding differences in value systems enhances a family's ability to communicate meaningfully and to share important decision-making activities. Affective primer exercises enable families to identify what is truly important in their past, current, and future patterns of relating to older members. Subsequently, problem areas may be renegotiated to assure continued development of the individual and family system. Affective primers aid intergenerational communication especially for the elderly who are more compressed by current psychosocial conditions than impaired.

Affect abilities training in various forms has been used for more impaired elderly. The few studies that have examined the issues concentrate largely on clinical research with significantly impaired elderly and have demonstrated positive outcomes (Filer & O'Connell, 1964). Activity and recreational programs in institutional settings are common and generally report positive results. The most systematic of these clinical approaches include reality orientation (Folsom, 1967), remotivation therapy (Dennis, 1976), validation therapy (Wetzler & Feil, 1979), remotivation as behavior therapy (Toepfer, Bicknell, & Shaw, 1974) and life review of reminiscence therapy (Kiernat, 1979). Generally, improvements in one area of functioning do not necessarily generalize to other areas of functioning; the gains manifest during the affective, reality-based therapy may not persist outside or after treatment (Lawton, 1980). Nonetheless, if changes in the affective content of the environment can bring about changes in a severely impaired person's level of competence, even if the change is situational, it is important to push the boundaries of this type of approach. The following description of recent clinical research may be helpful in boundary pushing.

Affect Abilities Training

The design of the exploratory affect abilities program was based on three assumptions: (1) that global cognitive changes associated with pathological aging interfere with the individual's ability to process affective information in natural settings; (2) that disruptive processing of affective elements underlies many problem behaviors; and (3) that affect training and practice with paying attention to individual and group feelings, expressing affective responses connected to a particular stimulus, valuing the dialogue relating the social events to past experiences that were valued by the self, and generalizing the event in relation to current world view would result in a decrease of negative social behaviors, improved satisfaction with the social exchange, and improved valuing of the self.

The intent of this research project was to explore the impact of affective training and practice on the socioemotional expressive behavior of older persons and staff in a community daycare setting and intermediate-care setting. Specifically, the clinical objectives were to bring about the following changes:

1. increase appropriate identification of emotional/affective states in self and others in the environment through specific affect abilities training
2. increase integration of past affective states into present environments, which may meaningfully reengage the individual's affective/motivational system
3. broaden the individual's interests/activities bands that are vehicles or targets for affective investment and expression
4. identify motivational aspects of affective expression and management aspects of affect in order for families and staff to bring about systematic and therapeutic change in affective responses

Eighteen subjects were recruited for the project, nine residing at an intermediate-care facility and nine attending a daycare program in the community. The level of impaired functioning based on clinical assessment reveals predictable differences in abilities between the two groups. The group attending the daycare program were relatively younger in age, ranging from 65 to 78 years, and had fewer physical ailments. The residents at the intermediate-care facility were older, ranging in age from 72 to 90 years, and exhibited major cognitive impairments.

A number of standardized instruments and project-designed instruments were used for collecting pre- and post-measures. The utility of the measuring probes varied in terms of obtaining meaningful individual performance measures; however, the instruments did provide a systematic approach for cognitive and affective skill sampling. Exhibit 4-2, the affect abilities checklist (Bell, Corcoran, Delaney, Kirchner, & Levinson, 1976), was used to elicit the staff's and family's view of the individual's affect abilities with four basic emotions and to guide the selection of training activities.

This checklist was frequently very tedious. Possible explanations include the novel nature of the task, resistance to identifying how an older person does

Exhibit 4–2 Affect Abilities Checklist

Staff/Family   Name _____

Site _____   Age _____

                                               Date _____
                                                    PRE, POST, POST

BASIC SKILLS   (NEVER) 1 2 3 4 5 (MOST OF THE TIME)

1. Demonstrates a knowledge of emotional words
     Anger _____
     Fear _____
     Sadness _____
     Happiness _____
2. Recognizes the emotional content of facial expressions
     Anger _____
     Fear _____
     Sadness _____
     Happiness _____
3. Recognizes the emotional content of physical gestures
     Anger _____
     Fear _____
     Sadness _____
     Happiness _____
4. Recognizes the emotional content of various bodily postures
     Anger _____
     Fear _____
     Sadness _____
     Happiness _____
5. Recognizes the emotional content in the tone of someone's voice
     Anger _____
     Fear _____
     Sadness _____
     Happiness _____
6. Recognizes the emotional content in the volume of someone's voice
     Anger _____
     Fear _____
     Sadness _____
     Happiness _____
7. Recognizes the emotional content in the pressure of someone's voice
     Anger _____
     Fear _____
     Sadness _____
     Happiness _____
8. Demonstrates an ability to express an emotion accurately
     Anger _____
     Fear _____
     Sadness _____
     Happiness _____
9. Demonstrates an ability to express emotion verbally
     Anger _____
     Fear _____

Sadness _____
Happiness _____

10. Demonstrates an ability to express emotion nonverbally
    Anger _____
    Fear _____
    Sadness _____
    Happiness _____

11. Expresses emotion within the bounds of social appropriateness
    Anger _____
    Fear _____
    Sadness _____
    Happiness _____

12. Demonstrates an ability to control his or her reactions to the emotions of others
    Anger _____
    Fear _____
    Sadness _____
    Happiness _____

13. Demonstrates an ability to effect an emotional response in others
    Anger _____
    Fear _____
    Sadness _____
    Happiness _____

14. Demonstrates an ability to respond empathetically to other persons
    Anger _____
    Fear _____
    Sadness _____
    Happiness _____

PROCESS SKILLS

15. Understands the causes of his or her emotions
    Anger _____
    Fear _____
    Sadness _____
    Happiness _____

16. Understands the effects of his or her emotions
    Anger _____
    Fear _____
    Sadness _____
    Happiness _____

17. Accepts his or her feelings
    Anger _____
    Fear _____
    Sadness _____
    Happiness _____

18. Understands the difference between his or her emotions and the emotions of others
    Anger _____
    Fear _____
    Sadness _____
    Happiness _____

19. Realizes when his or her verbal and nonverbal expressions of emotions don't match
    Anger _____

Fear _____
Sadness _____
Happiness _____
20. Recognizes his or her internal cues for emotions
    Anger _____
    Fear _____
    Sadness _____
    Happiness _____
21. Knows the difference between having an emotion and expressing it
    Anger _____
    Fear _____
    Sadness _____
    Happiness _____
22. If you were to ask the client how he or she felt, what kind of response   would
    you likely get?

    _____
    _____
    _____
    _____
    _____

Source: Adapted from *Affect Abilities Training: A Manual of Emotional Training and Psychotherapy for Low Intellectually Functioning Developmentally Disabled Persons* by B.A. Bell, J.R. Corcoran, R.J. Delaney, K.R. Kirchner, & W.S. Levinson. (Mimeographed.) Larimer County Mental Health Clinic, Department of Health, Education, and Welfare, Region 8, 1976. Reprinted with permission of K.R. Kirchner and R. Delaney, 1982.

really feel, and the general negative stereotyping that all older people are somewhat senile and emotionally constricted. Despite its tedious qualities, the checklist did serve as a good stimulus for discussion.

The group activities were designed by an educational therapist, and the groups were led by a gerospsychiatrist. While 480 minutes of intervention was scheduled, gathering everyone at a common location each session took 10 minutes or more. The inconsistency with which some subjects were able to participate further confounded the results. One subject died of heart disease, one was hospitalized, and several others refused to participate on different occasions. Training techniques were based on clinical experiences that suggested that (1) too often environments for impaired elderly are unstimulating and a range of objects and tasks can be used to enhance stimulation; (2) affective responses can be reinforced and expanded; (3) affect stimuli for specific individuals, once identified, can be recorded and recycled; and (4) knowing how and what stimulates a person enables the clinician to obtain a better picture of the affective domain of personal functioning and understanding of the personality.

The affective training activities were built around the concrete engagement of one or more senses, e.g., sight, smell, touch, feeling, hearing. For example, one session consisted of identifying the smell of items in glass containers, such as cloves, dill, cinnamon, soap, mothballs, and then encouraging individuals to talk about how these smells related to past experiences. As the group passed the containers and tried to determine the scent, a lively discussion ensued. It was clear that the concrete olfactory stimulus had activated memories filled with emotion. Another session used ripe tomatoes, which the group smelled and tasted; they then talked about harvesting and canning tomatoes. Every individual in the midwestern community had some experience with ripening tomatoes, which set the stage for group remembering—"once I had." The phrase *once I had* was then used as a stem for a group poem, with each individual contributing. The poem was typed and circulated at the next session and shared with the nursing staff.

Poetry proved to be very powerful and was used frequently in affect training. Photographs were also powerful stimuli for recalling past events. Instant snapshots of staff and group participants brought reminiscing based on old photos to the present. The changes in times, in families, and in one's self were reviewed. In all sessions, concrete material was used to activate participants. Familiar items from the past were used to motivate and enhance attentiveness. The group process was used to increase social relating on a very basic scale, such as wearing name tags and passing items from person to person, to more complex levels of social connecting. Lastly, the authors provided the associative stimuli by relating past and present experiences with stimuli and integrating current information about the self to past, present, and future expressions.

A direct result of the study appeared to be definition of the institutional or systems protectiveness of older people from exploration of the feeling function. There seemed to be an unspoken belief that the project would create disruption, conflict, and sadness if the older person began to express true feelings. This was displayed in a variety of ways with resistance in scheduling and staff support of individual avoidance of the group. This finding led to an expansion of the individual approach to a systems review of the interrelatedness of differing motivations, protectiveness, and investment in the status quo. It becomes clear that individuals' affective expression is part of the stable social milieu interaction. In addition to individual differences in discrimination, appreciation, expression, and range of feelings, there is also the environmental contribution to maintaining, enhancing, or promoting this.

An indirect or secondary "result" included a systems approach to feeling expression. Institutional environments create a restrictiveness of affective expression. For example, in a nursing home environment there are a limited number of ways to "feel." Negative or aggressive behaviors are interpreted as universally bad or pathological rather than legitimate. Positive affective behaviors are interpreted superficially as alertness. Expressed feelings are quickly and readily interpreted without expansion, further exploration, or connection to situation/precipitants due to the time and resource limitations of these environments.

The daycare environment included a variety of people representing differing diagnostic categories, levels of adjustment within the community, and individual personality styles. The subject who engaged in the research long enough to display adequate results or change was EL, a 73-year-old widow with obsessive-compulsive fault-finding patterns and a history of emotional trauma surrounding the abuse of alcohol and departure of her son five years prior to attempts at intervention. Through individual therapy, centered primarily around developing insight, she had displayed a great many affective resistances and defenses.

For these reasons, she was considered a good candidate for affective training to restructure her approach. She participated in the projects from a sense of duty, with consistent commitment and cooperation. She was able to develop some capacity to expand her affective range, which was evident to both group leaders and to other staff. The use of affective probing statements aided in the development of insight, as evidenced by her spontaneous comment, "I guess I was feelingless." She reported that early in life the family stimulated strong feeling and then in later life, the feeling "I hate to have people dislike me so." She reported in young adult and midadult life feelings about doing things perfectly—"housework," "duty"—and now in older life, "I couldn't care less."

Pretesting was difficult due to her disruptive emotional state; posttesting revealed extremes in feelings. Sample statements follow:

I am usually completely bored.
Life to me seems completely routine.
In life I have no goals or aims.
My personal existence is utterly meaningless, without purpose.
Every day is exactly the same.
If I could choose, I would prefer never to have been born.
My life is empty, filled only with despair.
If I should die today, I would feel that my life has been completely worthless.
As I view the world in relation to life, the world completely confuses me.
Concerning man's freedom to make his own decisions, I believe man is neutral.
With regard to suicide, I have thought of it seriously as a way out.

I regard my ability to find meaning, purpose, or mission in life as neutral.
My life is more out of my hands and controlled by external forces.
Facing my daily tasks is a painful and boring experience.
I have discovered no mission or purpose in life.

This study was unique in that it approaches an old organic population with habilitative techniques. The severely cognitively impaired population has not been studied for a variety of reasons, including the attention span of the population, the major confusion, and memory failures as well as a lack of clear approaches to managing behavior. The approach to exploring affect was valid throughout disruptions, verbal failures, and confusion. The process under investigation was never lost or changed—fluctuated yes, but not disrupted or lost. A positive outcome of these primitive efforts was that the attention of this group of 9—12 on occasion—was easily managed by 2 people despite the population's organic problems, memory deficits, language deficits, impulse control deficits, visual deficits, and social skill deficits.

The impact of this project on the system was positive in that it sensitized the staff to the fact something could be done to manage problem behaviors. The nursing home staff rallied around a second project of affective management with great interest and motivation. The immediate results of the group activities were evident to all staff members when the group was returned to the unit in a more pleasant, socially integrated, more talkative, outer-directed way, with subject matter with which to interact with the staff.

In summary, it is clear that problems of mood, affect, and emotion do lend themselves to systematic interventions. Affective primers may be employed by family members to heighten intergenerational understanding and shared communication. Affect abilities training suggests at least some possible points of affective interface between a visiting family and a seriously impaired older member. Families can stay "in touch" with even the more disabled aged if they apply these understandings to transactions and relational patterns.

MAINTAINING ROLE BALANCE AND FAMILY BOUNDARIES

Given the dynamics of life-span development, it is not surprising that family structures are constantly changing. Despite this change, clear family boundaries—who is inside or outside the system—must be maintained for healthy functioning of the members (Kantor & Lehr, 1975). Ambiguity of the boundaries can increase dysfunction in an already stressed family system. For example, Boss, McCubbin, and Lester (1979) observe that if a family member is perceived as psychologically present but is actually physically absent, the boundary is unclear. Similarly, if a member is physically present but because of impairments or disengagement, psychologically absent, boundary difficulties appear. Minuchin (1974) notes that for maximum functioning the boundaries of subsystems must be clearly recognizable and defined sufficiently to enable members to carry out their familial roles. "A parental subsystem that includes a grandmother or a parental child can function quite well so long as lines of responsibilities and authority are clearly drawn" (p. 54). Role reversals (filial crisis), isolation, and usurpation of family responsibility by service bureaucracies rather than "filial maturity" and participatory caregiving are major disruptors of boundaries in families with older members. Boss (1980) concludes that "the greater the boundary ambiguity at various developmental and normative junctures throughout the family life cycle, the higher the family and individual dysfunction" (p. 447).

Failure to resolve boundary problems keeps the family system at a high level of stress, causing secondary dysfunction in members, especially vulnerable older members. Often boundaries are restored through shifting tasks and role changes; however, in the case of an older member requiring intense support, role shifts can lead to *role overload* for one or more members, resulting in even more stress. If an older person must suddenly assume responsibility for all financial planning, maintenance of the home and auto, shopping and other daily living chores, and care of the compromised or impaired spouse, then role functions quickly become overloaded, leading to additional stresses that often precipitate a family crisis. The family as a unit begins to struggle with role clarity on practical and socioemotional levels.

Rapoport's (1963) work focuses on the critical developmental transition points in the family life cycle. A family either responds adaptively to these challenges and grows or it responds in a maladaptive fashion, leading to further deterioration of the system. The direction of adjustment affects the mental health of individual family members as well as the survival of the family system as a treatment/habilitative milieu. In order to meet the challenges of boundary maintenance, families must be helped to understand the developmental demands of particular members and be guided in shaping structural variations (role redefinitions) if they are to remain functionally intact.

The problem-solving styles of families have been studied by David Reiss and others. There appears to be significant variation in style along at least three dimensions: configuration, coordination, and closure. Reiss and Oliveri (1980) theorize that variations in these dimensions that influence definition of problems may be related to a family's adaptive capacity to psychological distress and other forms of stress. Their work does not specifically focus on older families; however, the analysis is still applicable.

Configuration has to do with a family's ability to determine subtle patterns in the problem-solving process. Reiss and Oliveri (1980) report that families who score high on configuration in laboratory-type problems also exhibit healthy perceptions and organization of the family's role in relation to the community and social networks. These families also exhibit organized mastery of activities of daily living and practice rituals that engage them into wider social groups outside the home. Households in which families score low on configuration are often disorganized in terms of daily living and disconnected from the larger community. They exhibit few bridges between household patterns and social practices. Consequently, family members cannot travel easily between the subsystem of the family and other social groups. Moreover, the lack of rituals and family traditions prohibits the development of "stability zones" for members in developmental transitions.

Families exhibiting high coordination typically solve problems in a sympathetic manner and coordinate planning and scheduling of daily activities (Reiss & Oliveri, 1980). Individuals within the family system "occupy the same experimental world" (Reiss & Oliveri, 1980, p. 436) and see themselves as part of a group with prescribed responsibilities and responsiveness. Closure is a dimension that reflects a family's tendency to delay final decisions by extension and an ability to tolerate higher degrees of ambiguity. Families who delay closure tend to be more invested and more open to input from larger numbers of extended kin according to Reiss and Oliveri (1980). Early closure families use rituals and family traditions to shape and pace daily and festive events.

Each of the dimensions of problem-solving style influence the families' stress responses. Families low in configuration tend to perceive themselves as victimized by stressful events. Families exhibiting high configuration perceive a connection between their responses and environmental demands; furthermore, they sense a mastery over many of life's challenges. They may engage in more information seeking and investigation in the early stages of decision making and tend to experience a greater sense of accomplishment once the problem is solved. In low-configuration families, outcomes are viewed as independent of action and due to chance, bad luck, and victimization. It is obvious that families vary along a continuum of configuration from high to low. However, the family's location along this continuum may be predictive of how members will go about solving the developmental problems of older members.

Still other families, because of coordination or lack of it, will exhibit even more diverse problem-solving skills and stress-reaction patterns. Coordination refers to solidarity and consistency of world view. Stressful events such as out-of-home-placement decisions are assumed to affect the whole system. Role prescriptions are clear, and individuals work to solve the problem in relation to others in the family. Consensus when reached is genuine. In contrast, low-coordination families seldom achieve true consensus and fail to see the interrelation or impact of stressful events on all members. Closure refers to a family's tendency to orient to the here and now of stressful events or to use past traditions and experiences in responding. Low-closure families prefer to routinize experiences (Aldous, 1971) while high-closure families are more open to risk and tolerate novel solutions better than low-closure families.

Stress then will impact families differently, depending on the way events are defined; problem-solving techniques will reflect the families' preferred patterns, configuration, coordination, and closure. Boundary maintenance and role balance also are probably influenced by these three dimensions.

Therefore, coping strategies for stressors surrounding problems in mood, memory, and behavior must be prescribed with individual differences in mind. Some families will be more stressed than others by the same event because of structured differences. Mental health then is a matter of adaptive balance between problem demands and optimal response patterns for individuals and individual families. Some families will seek more information from professionals, exhibit more cooperation between members, and delay decisions longer than other families. But, the three dimensions generally should be considered separately by professionals assisting the family in problem solving and decision making. Mismatches of professional support with the family's style will lead to additional stress on an overburdened family. Individual strengths and weaknesses of family systems must be taken into account in order to preserve optimal family functioning.

REFERENCES

Aldous, J. A framework for the analysis of family problem solving. In J. Aldous, T. Condon, R. Hill, M. Straus, & I. Tallman (Eds.), *Family problem solving: A symposium on theoretical, methodological and substantive concerns.* Hinsdale, Ill.: Dryden, 1971.

Baltes, P.B., & Labouvie, G.V. Adult development of intellectual performance: Description, explanation and modification. In C. Eisdorfer & M.D. Lawton (Eds.), *The psychology of adult development and aging.* Washington, D.C.: American Psychological Association, 1973.

Bayne, J.R.D. Environmental modification for the older person. *Gerontologist*, 1971, *11*, 314–317.

Bell, B.A., Corcoran, J.R., Delaney, R.J., Kirchner, K.R., & Levinson, W.S. *Affect abilities training: A manual of emotional training and psychotherapy for low intellectually functioning developmentally disabled persons.* Mimeographed. Larimer County, Colo.: Larimer County Mental Health Clinic Department of Health, Education, and Welfare, Region 8, 1976.

Boss, P.G. Normative family stress: Family boundary changes across the life-span. *Family Relations*, 1980, *29* (2), 445–450.

Boss, P.G., McCubbin, H.I., & Lester, G. The corporate executive wife's coping patterns in response to routine husband-father absence. *Family Process*, 1979, *18*, 79–86.

Botwinick, J. *We are aging.* New York: Springer Publishing Company, 1981.

Boxer, A.M., & Cohler, B.J. *Personal time orientations of intergenerational conflicts in three-generational families.* Paper presented at the 33rd Annual Scientific Meeting of the Gerontological Society, San Diego, Calif., November 21–25, 1980.

Brady, J.V. Emotion: Some conceptual problems and psychological experiments. In M.B. Arnold (Ed.), *Feelings and Emotions*. New York: Academic Press, 1970.

Buss, A. *Psychology: Man in perspective*. New York: John Wiley & Sons, 1973.

Butler, R.N. The life review: An interpretation of reminiscence in the aged. *Psychiatry*, 1963, *26*, 65–76.

Butler, R.N. Senility reconsidered: Treatment possibilities for mental impairments in the elderly. *Journal of the American Medical Association*, 1980, *224*, 259–263.

Cameron, P. Mood as an indicant of happiness: Age, sex, social class and situational differences. *Journal of Gerontology*, 1975, *30*, 216–224.

Carkhuff, R.R. *Helping and human relations* (Vols. 1 & 2). New York: Holt, Rinehart & Winston, 1969.

Carroll, K., & Costello, P.B. *An exercise in understanding*. Mimeographed. Minneapolis: Ebenezer Center for Aging, 1979.

Dennis, H. Remotivation therapy for the elderly: A surprising outcome. *Journal of Gerontological Nursing*, 1976, *2* (6), 28–30.

Diller, L. A model for cognitive retraining in rehabilitation. *The Clinical Psychologist*, 1976, *26*, 13–15.

Entin, A.D. The use of photographs and family albums in family therapy. In A.S. Gurman (Ed.), *Questions and answers in the practice of family therapy*. New York: Brunner/Mazel, 1981.

Erikson, E.H. *Insight and responsibility* (2nd ed). New York: W.W. Norton, 1964.

Filer, R.N., & O'Connell, D.D. Motivation of aging persons. *Journal of Gerontology*, 1964, *19*, 15–22.

Folsom, J.C. Intensive hospital therapy of geriatric patients. *Current Psychiatric Therapies*, 1967, *7*, 14–18.

Hauser, M.J. Cognition commands change. *Journal of Psychiatric Nursing and Mental Health Services*, 1981, *3*, 19–26.

Hoyer, W.J. Application of operant techniques to the modification of elderly behavior. *Gerontologist*, 1973, *13*, 18–22.

Hoyer, W.J., Mishara, B.L., & Reidel, R.G. Problem behaviors as operants: Applications with elderly individuals. *Gerontologist*, 1975, *15*, 452–456.

Kanfer, F.H., & Saslow, G. Behavior analysis: An alternative to diagnostic classification. *Archives of General Psychiatry*, 1965, *12*, 529–538.

Kantor, O., & Lehr, W. *Inside the family*. San Francisco: Jossey-Bass, 1975.

Kiernat, J.M. The use of life review activity with confused nursing home residents. *The American Journal of Occupational Therapy*, 1979, *33* (5), 306–310.

Krathwohl, D.R., Bloom, B.S., & Masia, B.B. Taxonomy of educational objectives. *Affective domain handbook II*. New York: David McKay, 1956.

Labouvie-Veiff, G., Hoyer, W.J., Baltes, M.M., & Baltes, P.B. Operant analysis of intellectual behavior in old age. *Human Development*, 1974, *17*, 259–272.

Lawson, R. Thirty years of research on the subjective well-being of older Americans. *Journal of Gerontology*, 1978, *33*, 109–125.

Lawton, M.P. Psychosocial and environmental approaches to the care of senile dementia patients. In J.O. Cole & J.E. Barrett (Eds.), *Psychopathology in the aged*. New York: Raven Press, 1980.

Liberman, R.P. Managing resistance to behavioral family therapy. In A.S. Gurman (Ed.), *Questions and answers in the practice of family therapy*. New York: Brunner/Mazel, 1981.

Maddox, G.L. Families as context and resource in chronic illness. In S. Sherwood (Ed.), *Long-term care.* New York: Spectrum Publications, 1975.

Meichenbaum, D. Self-instructional strategy training: A cognitive prosthesis for the aged. *Human Development,* 1974, *17,* 273-280.

Meichenbaum, D. *Cognitive behaviors modification.* New York: Plenum, 1977.

Meyer, A. The life chart. In Alfred Lief (Ed.), *The common sense psychiatry of Dr. R. Adolf Meyers.* New York: McGraw-Hill Book Company, 1948.

Minuchin, S. *Families and family therapy.* Cambridge: Harvard University Press, 1974.

Neugarten, B. Acting one's age: New rules for old. *Psychology Today,* April 1980, pp. 66-80.

Neugarten, G.L. Time, age and the life cycle. *American Journal of Psychiatry,* 1979, *136,* 887-894.

Piaget, J. *The construction of reality in the child.* New York: Basic Books, 1954.

Rapoport, R. Normal crises, family structure and mental health. *Family Process,* 1963, 2 (1), 68-80.

Rebok, G.W., & Hoyer, W.J. The functional context of elderly behavior. *Gerontologist,* 1977, *17,* 27-34.

Reisberg, B., & Ferris, S.H. Diagnosis and assessment of the older patient. *Hospital and Community Psychiatry,* 1982, *33* (2), 104-110.

Reiss, D., & Oliveri, M.E. Family paradigm and family coping: A proposal for linking the family's intrinsic adaptive capacities to its responses to stress. *Family Relations,* 1980, *29* (4), 431-444.

Riegel, K.F., & Reigel, R.M. Development, drop and death. *Developmental Psychology,* 1972, *6,* 306-319.

Schaie, W.K. Psychological changes from mid life to early old age: Implication for the maintenance of mental health. *American Journal of Orthopsychiatry,* 1981, *51,* 199-218.

Schultz, R. Emotionality and aging: A theoretical and empirical analysis. *Journal of Gerontology,* 1982, *37* (1), 42-51.

Seligman, M.E. *Helplessness.* San Francisco: W.H. Frieman, 1975.

Smith, L., & Gray-Feiss, K. *Memory development: An approach for responding to the mentally impaired elderly in the long-term care setting.* Paper presented at the 30th Annual Scientific Meeting of the Gerontological Society, San Francisco, November 1977.

Toepfer, C.T., Bicknell, A.T., & Shaw, D.O. Remotivation as behavior therapy. *Gerontologist,* 1974, *14,* 451-453.

Weinberg, J. What do I say to my mother when I have nothing to say? *Geriatrics,* 1974, *29,* 155-159.

Wetzler, M.A., & Feil, N. *Validation therapy with disoriented aged who use fantasy. Manual.* Cleveland: Edward Feil Productions, 1979.

Zarit, S.H. *Aging and mental disorders.* New York: Free Press, 1980.

Zepelin, H., Wolfe, C.S., & Kleinplatz, F. Evaluation of a year long reality orientation. *Journal of Gerontology,* 1981, *36* (1), 70-77.

Chapter 5

Scope of Concerns

A wide range of specific concerns emerges from the complex psychological lives of older people. Individual processes for identifying these concerns are as unique and varied as older individuals themselves. Some specific concerns are intuited; others are anticipated due to attitudes, prejudices, and role expectation of our culture; yet others are identified and experienced through the direct involvement with older peers, spouses, and loved ones. Family members likewise have a variety of methods for identifying specific concerns among their older members. Professionals and aging workers have a responsibility to evaluate these specific concerns. The process of evaluation, however, is multileveled. The challenge becomes matching the correct level of evaluation with the level of pathology or distress. General screening, which a health maintenance clinic provides, may be appropriate for minor distresses. Other general concerns may require complete assessment while specific major concerns may require intensive, specific assessments.

Case finding has emerged as an attempt to find older people with specific concerns and match them with the appropriate level of evaluation. Case finding for specific psychological distresses must cover a wide range of areas and disciplines. Many cases can be found in general health clinics due to the high frequency of older distressed individuals presenting for medical evaluation and treatment. The infrequent presentation of older distressed individuals to mental health clinics or psychiatric services is widely recognized. Case finding in social settings such as nutrition sites, senior centers, and church and community groups has potential; however, a nagging question always remains, What frail, distressed older person isn't here?

The process of professional involvement in elaborating and specifically defining concerns is variegated and subject to a history of biases and prejudices (Butler, 1975a). As outlined in earlier chapters, the concept of functional capacity is important and serves as an integrative focus for specific problem identification and solution; however, it suffers from a lack of comprehensive

123

application by the service community. Butler (1968) defines another challenge to professionals when he emphasizes the need for a form of paleopsychiatry to understand specific concerns of the individual against the backdrop of sociocultural change.

Psychiatric involvement with older people has been largely restricted to diagnostic assessment. Consequently, the current psychiatric interview falls short by not including integrative life-span histories and uncovering the full meaning of psychological distresses of aging. Studies of attitudes of psychiatrists toward the aged reveal consistent findings of bias, limited treatment objectives, and noticeable lack of focus on the clinical challenges of psychiatric care for older people. Butler and Lewis (1982) acknowledge these challenges and have identified a personal data-screening instrument of wide range and focus for use in sifting through specific concerns of older people in psychiatric settings. Reiff (1980) likewise has proposed the need for a life medical history of specific medical concerns across the life span.

Modification of Meyer's (1948) life chart may also be extremely useful in initial screening of presenting problems of older members (see Chapter 4). Meyer's original life chart provides a common-sense view of the life span and advocates a provisional thought pattern based on the endless detail and variety across the life span. The life chart was used to integrate important data about the patient in chronological order from birth to the future. The life chart forms a tracing of the life curve of the entire organism. The life chart also defines the level of integration of the organism in relationship to its environment and begins to define the record of development and condition of the integrated personality. Meyer systematically recorded date of birth and age with subsequent situations and reactions surrounding biological events. The approach has been expanded by the authors to include a biopsychosocial life event approach as depicted in Figure 5–1, the biopsychosocial life chart.

The biopsychosocial life chart begins to outline the specific concerns of older members and their families. Older individuals sense that they are in higher risk categories for physical ailments such as heart disease, arthritis, and stroke as well as the higher risk categories for cognitive impairments and the functional impairments of depression, paranoia, and anxiety. The multiple threats to the biopsychosocial integrity of the personality increase the urgency of understanding a specific concern.

The aging worker must have a keen sense of the frequent concerns of older people. Early warning signs of distress and potential escalation of distress must be appreciated. The degree of distress must be understood. Minor problems must be separated from major concerns; mild distress must be differentiated from disease; typical change must be distinguished from life-threatening change.

Figure 5-1 Biopsychosocial Life Chart

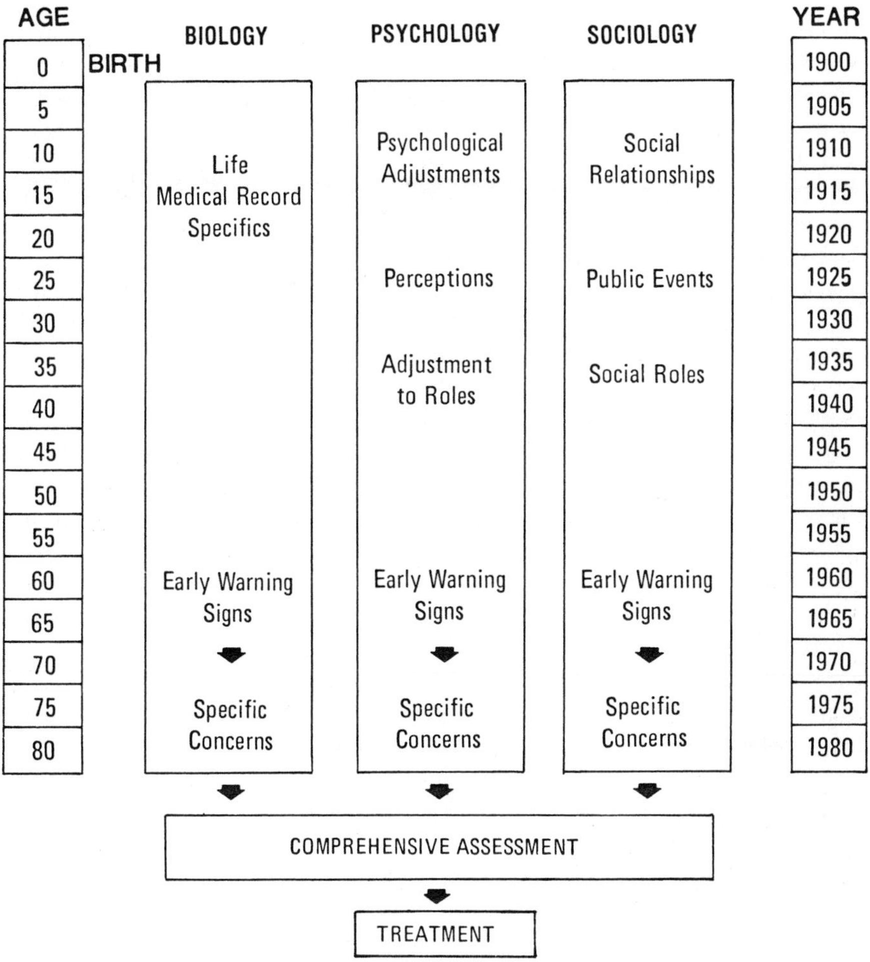

AGE	BIOLOGY	PSYCHOLOGY	SOCIOLOGY	YEAR
0	BIRTH			1900
5				1905
10	Life	Psychological Adjustments	Social Relationships	1910
15	Medical Record			1915
20	Specifics			1920
25		Perceptions	Public Events	1925
30				1930
35		Adjustment to Roles	Social Roles	1935
40				1940
45				1945
50				1950
55				1955
60	Early Warning Signs	Early Warning Signs	Early Warning Signs	1960
65				1965
70	⬇	⬇	⬇	1970
75	Specific Concerns	Specific Concerns	Specific Concerns	1975
80				1980

⬇ ⬇ ⬇

COMPREHENSIVE ASSESSMENT

⬇

TREATMENT

This chapter briefly reviews specific psychological concerns frequently identified by older people and their families. The processes for evaluation of specific concerns that become psychological distresses or clear and manifest psychiatric disorders are outlined. Specific problems of differential diagnosis, etiology, and current recommended treatments are reviewed for specific problems associated with cognitive impairments, psychiatric disorders, functional disorders, alcoholism, and physical ailments.

COGNITIVE IMPAIRMENTS

The threat and reality of cognitive impairments with increasing age are a major concern of older people and their families. The extent of cognitive impairments is clear in the reported incidence among older people. Approximately 10 percent of individuals over 65 years of age are estimated to have clinically significant cognitive impairments (NIA, 1980). The percentage increases to 20 percent by age 80. From 50 to 75 percent of nursing home residents suffer major cognitive impairments. The most common specific type of cognitive impairment alone, primary degenerative dementia, is recognized as the fourth leading cause of death (Katzman, 1976). With the magnitude of this problem, it is not surprising that most older people have had some exposure to the destructiveness of cognitive impairments of their peers, relatives, friends, or selves. This exposure and a continued socialization to expect "senility" with increasing age (Butler, 1975b) create a highly charged emotional concern.

Families and their older members sense that cognitive impairments represent a frequent and profound challenge to healthy aging. Cognitive abilities are intimately related to definition of self and total functioning as well as achievement of the late-life developmental tasks of maintenance of dignity, self-esteem, and a sense of purpose and belonging. The context of the older individual's self is disrupted and distorted in subtle and insidious ways by cognitive impairments.

Cognitive impairments among older people present a complex symptomatology and behavior change, a multiplicity of causes, and a poorly defined natural progression. Minor cognitive declines with age are generally accepted as typical. However, the challenge lies in separating typical age-related changes from early pathological changes, differentiating reversible changes from irreversible changes, and accurately determining the cause of impairments.

The degrees of cognitive impairment can perhaps be usefully viewed for a moment on an artificial continuum. Mild degrees of impairment such as benign senescent forgetfulness usually include minor memory failures and sometimes delays in recall. Moderate degrees of impairment such as the confusional states of reversible dementias and delirium include fluctuations in mental functioning with resulting behavior changes. Major degrees of impairment such as the later stages of irreversible dementias involve major disruptions of basic cognitive processing of personal and environmental details. The resulting disorientation, major memory failure, and judgment impairments totally disrupt the function of the personality. It is imperative that every effort be made to explore the degree of impairment and its cause regardless of the position along the continuum at the time of presentation.

In an effort to unravel the complexity of cognitive impairments and change with age, researchers and academicians have focused attention on adult cognitive development and processing. With this increasing interest in cognition and the complete life span, limitations of earlier cognitive developmental models such as Piaget's have become more apparent (Flavell, 1970; Piaget, 1972). Theorists are left with the conceptual challenge of extending cognitive development theory to the entire life span given a sizable knowledge base accumulated in the individual components of cognitive processing. Basic research on cognition and aging has largely been limited to the individual components of intelligence and memory. More recent attention has focused on problem solving, language, social relationships, and adaptive capacity or plasticity of the cognitive processing system. Further information is needed about the influences of life experience, education, vocational achievements, social opportunities, and motivation on the cognitive processing of older people.

The question of changing intellectual abilities with aging has been vigorously explored. Many issues remain unexplained (Botwinick, 1967); the polarity of research findings ranges from decline of intellectual capacity with age to change in intellectual capacity with age, not necessarily decline. The controversy over intellectual decline is complicated by a number of factors, including research methodology, sampling techniques, and basic definitions of intelligence. Baltes and Schaie (1974) emphasize little or no decline in intellectual function with age.

Despite vigorous exploration of memory function and aging, many questions about this component of cognition also remain unanswered. Basic hypotheses explaining memory decline are being challenged by hypotheses that appear more relevant to the aging experience (Burke & Light, 1981). Researchers are beginning to broaden the understanding of memorial processes and explore what an older person is able to say about his or her memory ability.

A wide range of information must be integrated from research and academic sources for use in understanding the complex nature of cognitive changes in older people. A biopsychosocial information-processing matrix is useful in systematic organization of this information (Rich & Eyde, 1981). Information processing consists of information input through the perceptual processes, information processing or storage, and information output or retrieval. These components are summarized in biological, psychological, and social areas in Table 5-1.

Biological factors that affect information input include visual loss, hearing loss, and energy level, which may be decreased by normal aging, diseases, or medications. Biological factors that affect processing and output include nerve cell loss, neurotransmitter changes, strokes, and dementias.

Psychological factors that affect information input include cautiousness, motivation, attention mechanisms, attitude, interest and affective states such as depression. Psychological factors that influence information processing include the meaningfulness of information, amount of practice, and use of the mecha-

Table 5-1 Cognitive Matrix

	INPUT	PROCESSING	OUTPUT
BIOLOGICAL	Visual loss Hearing loss Energy level	Dementias Strokes Nerve cell loss Neurotransmitter changes	Dementias Strokes Nerve cell loss Neurotransmitter changes
PSYCHOLOGICAL	Cautiousness Attention Motivation Attitude Interest Affective state	Meaningful Practice Selective forgetting	Life review Self criticism Performance anxiety
SOCIAL	Retirement Age segregation Mobility and transportation problems Financial limitations	Minimal expectations Lack of social role for older learner	Lack of value for wisdom of aged

nism of selective forgetting. Psychological factors that influence information output include performance anxiety with the retrieval task, a self-critical approach, and the positive or negative values of life review.

Social factors affecting information processing are less widely appreciated. However, social factors that affect information input include age segregation of older people, which isolates them from mainstream information, and retirement, which isolates people from information in the work world. Additional factors are changes in mobility and lack of transportation, which limit participation in social activities, and financial limitations, which interfere with entertainment and activities that represent information input. The major social factor influencing information output is a lack of appreciation or value for the cognitive production or wisdom of older people.

Assessment of Cognitive Impairment

Assessment of cognitive impairments of older people begins when someone pays attention to the cognitive production and processing of older people and questions change. Families express a variety of concerns as they observe minor memory failures such as failure of name recall, misplaced object, or missed appointment. Repetition, rambling, general irritability, and delays in recall also concern families. Cognitive impairments often appear gradually with only subtle changes. Consequently, families and spouses may gradually assume decision-making demands, readjust cognitive demands, and compensate for changes in functions without question. Unfortunately, many families do not assist their cognitively impaired older members to seek help. Often clinicians evaluate dementias in middle and later stages. Impaired individuals rarely present themselves for evaluation, though in early stages there is often a subjective distress. Older people may be affected by a defensiveness about their education or cognitive abilities. Many are self-depreciating about their incomplete educations. Many sense different cognitive styles, which they equate with diminished abilities.

The complexity of symptoms, causes, and resistances to assessment demand further community education and sensitivity on the part of workers with the aging. Families and older people must be directed to complete assessments when cognitive change and impairment are sensed. The family's role in complete assessment is not widely appreciated but is clearly sensed by experienced clinicians. Cognitive impairments contribute to inaccurate and incomplete histories. The defense of denial may interfere with accurate identification of functional impairments or problems as a result of cognitive impairments. These gaps can be filled by involved family members, usually a spouse. Basic questions that must be answered in complete assessments include the cause of impairment, extent of impairment, resulting behavioral changes, adaptive capacity, and functional capacity, including-self care and the ability to meet environmental demands.

Complete evaluation of cognitive impairments must include a history, physical examination, and the following battery of tests: serum enzymes and electrolytes, blood-urea-nitrogen (BUN), creatinine, glucose, complete blood cell count, urinalysis, chest X-ray, serological test for syphilis, thyroid function studies, vitamin B12 and folate levels, and computerized axial tomography of the brain (Wells, 1979). This represents a minimum battery necessary to diagnose any potential reversible cause of delirium or dementia. Additional testing may be indicated by abnormalities in the physical examination or suspicions raised in the history. Further psychological testing may be useful in distinguishing depressive cognitive changes from other forms of cognitive impairments

(Wells, 1977; Klisz, 1978). Several assessments may be necessary to follow the extent of impairment and rate of decline or recovery.

A number of screening instruments are helpful in initial documentation of major cognitive impairments. These include the mini-mental state (Folstein, Folstein, & McHugh, 1975), short portable mental status (Pfeiffer, 1975), FROMAJE—a mental status evaluation of function, reasoning, orientation, memory, arithmetic, judgment, and emotional state—(Libow, 1977), and the mental status questionnaire (Kahn, Goldfarb, Pollack, & Peck, 1960). They all have general application and test the basics of cognitive function: orientation, memory, reasoning, calculations, etc. Some are helpful in determining the extent of impairment. These instruments, however, must be integrated with history, physical examination, and a more complete mental status evaluation with particular attention to possible depression, psychotic thinking, and aphasias or focal neurological deficits.

Adaptive capacity can be clinically interpreted from behavior observation of the person's response to cognitive demands as well as interaction with the interviewer. Rich and Eyde (1980) have described a framework for organizing components of insight and adaptive responses of cognitively impaired elderly. Common adaptations of information-processing skills are increased use of external storage, practice or repetition. Increased awareness of limited capacity and conservation of energy result in distancing and avoidance of cognitive demands. Common affective adjustments include obvious anxiety and frustration, a hostile or defensive posturing, depression or withdrawal, and occasionally swings from combative-confusion to passive-compliance. Adaptive responses that are apparent with great individual variation include direct avoidance of the cognitive demands; substitution of comfortable, familiar subjects to avoid cognitive demands; repetition; and complete surrender and withdrawal.

Differential Diagnosis

Benign forgetfulness and pseudodementia are critical issues in the accurate diagnosis of cognitive impairments of older people. Kral (1978) describes benign senescent forgetfulness, a condition occurring with increasing frequency with age, though not progressive. Characteristics of this memory impairment include impaired recall for relatively unimportant information as well as parts of experiences and occasional delays in recall. This is considered a normal age-related change and must be differentiated from more malignant and progressive impairments.

The issue of pseudodementia or depressive illness that presents a clinical picture similar to dementia is more complex. Kiloh (1961) initially described the phenomenon, which has captured increasing clinical interest. The differentiation of depression and dementia is further complicated by the reported high incidence of depression associated with dementia (Post, 1962; Ernst, Badask, Beran, Kosovsky, & Kleinhauz, 1977). Furthermore, memory complaint has been related to the level of depression regardless of performance (Kahn, Zarit, Hilbert, & Niederehe, 1975).

In the area of treatment, Sternberg and Jarvik (1976) show an improvement in the short-term memory deficits of depressed individuals treated with antidepressant medications. Miller (1980) systematically explored mood and cognitive impairments among older people and made a surprising conclusion. Despite the high incidence of sustained and genuine depressive symptoms among cognitively impaired elderly, very few were treated for depression. The complexity of diagnosing early dementia and the atypical presentation of depressions in older people create a major clinical challenge and fear of misdiagnosis. Duckworth and Ross (1975) point out that U.S. clinicians diagnose dementia more frequently and depression less frequently than Canadian or United Kingdom clinicians. This suggests that individual characteristics of clinicians influence this diagnostic dilemma.

History and examination are important for accurate differential of dementia, depression, and dementia with depression. Raskind and Storrie (1980) state that a careful history of the development of the illness is most useful. The onset of depression includes dysphoric mood, loss of interest, decreased energy and activity, changes in appetite and sleep, impaired concentration, and increased somatic complaints. The onset of dementia includes memory failures, decreased attention, confabulation, and perseveration. Differences in response to examination are evident. The depressed individual appears to suffer from a motivation problem and withdraws from cognitive demands. The demented individual suffers from performance anxieties and may develop a catastrophic reaction of increased agitation and avoidance when cognitive demands are presented. Kiloh (1961) suggests that pseudodementia should be considered when an individual presents with a recent onset of a demented appearance with a normal EEG. When in doubt, depressive features should be treated and patients followed closely to monitor change.

Reversible causes of cognitive impairments account for 10 to 20 percent of all cognitive impairments in persons over 65 years of age (Wells, 1978; Marsden & Harrison, 1972). It is extremely important to explore aggressively and eliminate these conditions whenever possible in order to prevent further deterioration. The most common causes of reversible impairments are therapeutic drug intoxications, depression, a variety of metabolic diseases, and infections. Other causes include heart diseases such as congestive heart failure, acute myocardial infarcts, or arrhythmias. Malnutrition is also a common cause of confusion, which is reversible with diet correction. Additional impairments are brain disorders such as stroke, head trauma, subdural hematomas, epidural hematomas, brain infections, tumors, or normal pressure hydrocephalus. Other causes of reversible cognitive impairments include pain, sensory deprivation, and hospitalization or change in surrounding (NIA, 1980).

The irreversible causes of cognitive impairment include the dementias: primary degenerative dementia or Alzheimer's disease, multiple infarct dementia, alcoholic dementia, Parkinson's dementia, and a diverse group of less common dementias. Dementias are characterized by progressive and global deteriorations in memory, comprehension, abstraction, judgment, orientation, and emotional responsiveness and control. Other terms frequently used to describe dementias include *chronic organic brain syndrome* and *organic mental syndrome.*

Primary degenerative dementia of the Alzheimer's type represents the most common form of dementia. The onset is insidious, with a progressive deterioration in cognitive function, behavior, adaptation, and function. The incidence increases with age; the average age of onset is 74 (Wang & Whanger, 1971). Life expectancy is shortened, and most deaths are attributed to immediate causes such as heart failure or pneumonia.

Stages of the disease have recently been described and are helpful in understanding the natural progression and change in care needs (Mace & Rabins, 1982; Schneck, Reisberg, & Ferris, 1982). Stage 1 is described as forgetfulness, with memory failures for names, recent events, object placement, and appointments. Anxiety and subjectively reported distress may be apparent. Victims may try to adapt by increasing use of external storage, by writing things down, or by enlisting the help of other people in remembering.

Stage 2 is described as the confusional stage, with increasing memory failure, disorientation, and impaired concentration. Impulsiveness, hyperactivity, and social regression may be apparent. Problems with expressive speech and understanding may increase.

Stage 3 is the dementia stage. Cognitive functioning is severely impaired, with disorientation, behavioral problems, motor restlessness, and possible psychotic symptoms or paranoia, delusions, and hallucinations.

The cause of Alzheimer's disease is not known. However, the cellular pathology is clearly nerve cell loss and dysfunction. Possible explanations for the disease include viral infections (Sigurdsson, 1954), aluminum accumulation (Klatzo, Wisniewski, & Streicher, 1965), immune system defect (Tkach & Hokama, 1970), genetic inheritance (Constantinidis, 1978), and cholinergic system deficiency (Davies, 1978).

Multiple infarct dementia represents the second most common form of dementia. The onset, in contrast to Alzheimer's disease, is usually abrupt, with uneven deterioration. The average age of onset is 66. Often it is associated with the risk factors for cerebral vascular diseases: hypertension, diabetes mellitus, smoking, heart disease, and transient ischemic attacks (Reisberg & Ferris, 1982). The pathology is cerebral softenings as a result of repeated cerebral infarcts (Tomlinson, Blessed, & Roth, 1970; Jellinger, 1976).

Wernicke-Korsakoff's psychosis represents the most widely accepted dementia associated with alcoholism. There is, however, diagnostic confusion with other proposed diagnoses of alcoholic deterioration, alcoholic dementia, and subacute alcoholic encephalopathy (Wells, 1982). Alcohol has a direct neurotoxic effect on the brain. Malnutrition—especially thiamine deficiency—head trauma, and liver failure are also related to brain damage associated with alcoholism. The usual presentation of chronic cognitive impairment associated with alcoholism is that of impaired memory and attentional abilities that are often stable rather than progressive.

Parkinson's disease is associated with dementia in one-third of Parkinson's cases (Sweet, McDowell, & Feigenson, 1976; Lieberman, Dziatolowsky, & Kupersmith, 1979). This association is not well understood but tends to occur in older patients with a rapid and progressive decline.

Other less common causes of cognitive impairments include Pick's disease, which is clinically difficult to differentiate from Alzheimer's disease, and Creutzfeldt-Jakob disease, which involves a rapidly progressive decline associated with movement disorders.

Treatment of Cognitive Impairments

Theoretical approaches to the treatment of cognitive impairments, especially the dementias, are noticeably lacking. This may not be surprising given the lack of definitive understanding about the causes of these conditions. However, families and individuals suffer, and treatment efforts must be made. Treatment considerations must include more than biological treatment of the disease itself, for effective biological cures, suppression, or controls of the disease do not exist. Treatment must be directed at facilitating the psychological adjustment of the individual and his or her family; minimizing adverse psychological reactions such as agitation, depression, and paranoia; and improving the individual's interaction with his or her environment. Furthermore, the demented individual may have additional chronic or acute illnesses that contribute to impaired function; these must be diagnosed and treated.

Hollister (1981) is optimistic about continued research aimed at treatment despite a lack of definitive cause. He advocates combinations of new biological approaches rather than assuming that single-treatment trials will provide the answers. Crook and Gershon (1981) provide an excellent review of a variety of biological approaches.

Psychological approaches to the treatment of the dementias include a variety of theoretical formulations. Goldfarb (1967) proposes enhancing the natural dependencies of the cognitively impaired within an individual therapy relationship. Verwoerdt (1981) points out the importance of maintaining an optimal attitude and a realistic and consistent approach as well as getting and staying in touch with impaired older people in individual psychotherapy relationships. He further outlines specific treatment goals of early recognition and correction of associated psychosocial stress, adaptation of the environment to the patient, reduction of the patient's need for his or her impaired capacities, restitution and replacement of impaired function, maintenance and utilization of residual functions, and treatment of distress.

Brody, Kleban, Lawton, and Silverman (1971) studied the effect of individualized treatment plans on the excess disabilities of a group of mentally impaired aged. Their findings indicate a potential for improvement when an individual's unique traits, personality, history, and potential strengths are utilized. Other group approaches to treatment such as reality orientation, validation therapy, and memory development are discussed in Chapter 4.

Understanding the unique ways a cognitively impaired individual approaches and responds to the environment is vital to effective management of the dementias. Memory models depicting short-term memory deficits have been largely ineffective in creating a clearer understanding. Dementias clearly affect the short-term or working memory, making new learning or processing impossible or incomplete. Long-term memory stores are also affected in later stages of dementia; however, little is understood about the effect of long-term memory itself in the dementias. Reactivation of past experiences and memories must serve some function for cognitively impaired older people, given the frequency of reminiscing and past-directed discussions. Innate or automatic approaches to the environment are apparent when observing cognitively impaired individuals in familiar as well as novel environments. They appear to be making basic decisions about the environment such as safe or unsafe, familiar or unfamiliar, pleasant or unpleasant, old or new. These basic approaches appear deeply seated in the innate primitive processing mechanism and appear to influence behavior; however, this process is poorly understood.

Figure 5–2 presents a memory model for cognitive impairments and integrative therapy, which is useful in understanding the short-circuiting mechanisms operating in cognitively impaired elderly. When short-term memory deficits disrupt sequential reality based interaction with the environment, external psychosocial prosthetics must be provided. Integrative therapy presented in Chapter 4 summarizes an approach that facilitates activation of the sensory register, motivation to engage in further processing, habilitation of techniques and controls that substitute for short-term deficits, resonation of past experience lying dormant but available in the long-term memory stores, and integration into the present sensory environment.

Figure 5-2 Memory Model for Cognitive Impairment and Integrative Therapy

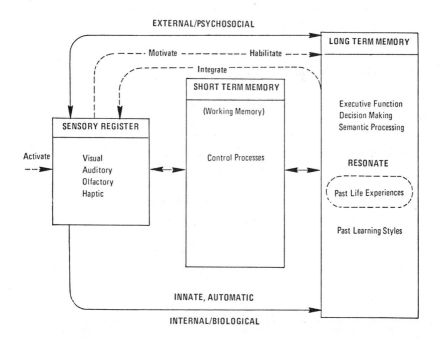

The family role in the treatment of the dementias has recently received more attention. LaBarge (1981) reviews counseling for families and points out the benefits to family and dementia patients. Brody (1977) points out the central role of the family in maximizing patient adaptation.

Treating the stressed family of a dementia victim requires special consideration. Hausmann (1979) points out the importance of dealing with initial grief and anger. Families must have help in assuming the caretaker role, balancing responsibilities, and setting realistic courses of action. In the early stages of dementia, families must pay attention to maintaining legal and financial security. The middle-stage responsibilities include providing a protected environment and psychological support. The third stage requires more care, often nursing home care, where family and staff must maintain the dignity and identity of the individual who can't do this alone (Mace & Rabins, 1982). Respite care is vitally important for the family (Weiler & Rathbone-McCuan, 1978). Medications for control of anxiety, agitation, and depression may be useful.

The treatment of the dementias is not a simple, singular task but requires the cooperation of many resources, family, and patient. While overall successes are limited, minor successes along the course of a progressive destructive disease are well worth the effort. Hopefully, future research will positively affect the prevention, diagnosis, and treatment of these devastating conditions.

PSYCHIATRIC DISORDERS

The magnitude of human suffering in psychiatric disorders of late life makes early identification of psychiatric warning signs extremely important. However, Lowenthal, Berkman, and associates (1967) have shown that behavior change of older people that is not physically harmful to self or others is often ignored for long periods. Further obstacles to effective identification and management of psychiatric disorders include a complex diagnostic dilemma for disorders of later life and a wide range of contributing biopsychosocial dysfunctions interpreted as normal. Commonly observed disorders of depression, anxiety, and paranoia are reviewed.

Depression

Depression is a common psychiatric disorder of late life, with an estimated 30 to 50 percent of people over age 65 suffering from a depressive episode severe enough to interfere with function (Ban, 1978). Depression represents the major cause of psychiatric hospitalization for older people. Depressive illnesses are often associated with incapacitating diseases (Dovenmuehle & Verwoerdt, 1963); this fact appears to influence their appropriate and timely treatment. Unfortunately, depressions in late life are often viewed as normative because of their association with physical diseases, cognitive impairments, metabolic disorders, and hypochondriasis, which in turn are mistakenly viewed as normative (Epstein, 1976).

Exploration of age differences in incidence, symptoms, or types of depression reveal few significant differences between depressions of the young and depressions of the old. Gurland (1976) discusses methodological problems in a study of these age-related differences. Winokur, Morrison, Clancy, and Crowe (1973) explored symptomatology and found no striking differences but note that agitation is more frequent in older depressives and retardation is more common in younger depressives. In regard to the course of the disease, Winokur (1974) found that chronic disease is more frequent in females over 40 years of age and recurrence is seen more frequently in men over 40. Few reliable data are available on age differences in the type of depression, but Mendlewicz (1976) makes a very practical observation that an early age of onset of depression is more positively correlated with a family history for depressive illness and implies a genetic predisposition. Late-onset depression then may be more closely related to environmental factors.

Symptoms of late-life depression then are similar to depressions of early life and involve depressed affect, crying, psychomotor agitation or retardation, vegetative signs of insomnia, decreased appetite, decreased weight, decreased sexual interest, constipation, fatigue, and muscle tension. Psychological symptoms of confusion, hopelessness, helplessness, irritability, impaired concentration, self-depreciation, ruminations, and suicidal thoughts may also be apparent. These symptoms may appear at varying rates and with different immediate precipitants. Symptoms may be successfully masked by some older individuals. On a practical level, measurements of degrees of depression may be useful. The functional assessment instrument of Chapter 3 is useful in documenting how and to what degree depression influences and depresses activities of daily living.

Another useful measure of depression involves assessment of degrees of social behavioral deficits. Social withdrawal is a common result of depressive feelings with concurrent psychological changes of lower self-esteem, increased irritability, and guilt feelings. Degrees of social withdrawal evident in the social communication process fall along the following continuum of increasing loss of social connectedness: normal speech, less spontaneous speech, less intimate speech, no spontaneous speech, constriction of all communicative responses, use of symbolic or idiosyncratic language, only "yes" or "no" answers, unintelligible verbal responses, only nonverbal responses, no eye contact, and passive or active avoidance of communication. Families can often describe their frustration with the restrictive communication of a depressed older member.

Evaluation of depression in the elderly must result in an effective treatment plan. Basic treatment differences require that depressions be separated into either reactive or biochemical types. Reactive depressions result from reaction to losses and are usually treated with psychotherapy. Biochemical depressions are related to theorized biochemical changes in neurotransmitters, usually do not have clear precipitants, and are treated with antidepressant medications. The distinction, however, is complicated by the serial losses of older people. Engel (1962) describes the following losses that contribute to depression in older people: (1) loss of loved person, (2) loss of health, (3) loss of job and social role, (4) loss of valued personal possessions, (5) changes in life style, (6) failure of lifelong plans or ventures, (7) loss of membership or status, and (8) loss of pets. Biochemical depressions are more frequently associated with the vegetative signs of depression and positive family histories for depression. In addition to different treatments for reactive or biochemical types of depression, treatment of depression in the elderly should be directed at all biopsychosocial dysfunctional areas.

A comprehensive review of each area in light of the symptoms is required to treat depression successfully. Biological issues that contribute to and cause depression are the biochemical imbalances in the neurotransmitters, as discussed. Certain diseases of the elderly may mimic depression, notably hypothyroidism. Several commonly used drugs can create a biochemical imbalance in neurotransmitters that results in depressivelike symptoms. These drugs include reserpine, hydrolazine, and methyldopa used for hypertension and procainamide and propranolal used for heart disease. Chronic diseases can also deplete energy reserves and create apathy or immobility that must be differentiated from depression.

Psychological issues that contribute to depression are losses that have been described. Other contributing factors include loss of self-esteem, repressed anger, bereavement, loss of emotional security, failed developmental transitions, and learned helplessness as described by Seligman (1975). Social issues that influence depression include loss of status, loss of social supports, and loss of financial security.

Psychologically oriented treatment can be used effectively and creatively by the treatment team. Most commonly used psychotherapies include individual supportive or insight-oriented psychotherapy. Commonly used group psychotherapies include supportive, insight-oriented, and family psychotherapies. The social therapies of milieu therapy, environmental manipulation, and occupational and recreational therapies are also useful. Treatment goals are to help the older person understand the nature of his or her illness, adjust to aging, and manage stress through reestablishing self-esteem and self-reliance.

Biological treatments include several categories of antidepressant medications, tricyclics, and monoamine oxidase inhibitors. Antidepressant medications work over a period of time, and results may not be apparent for two to four weeks. The usual adequate trial period is considered one month. Dosages for older people must be carefully monitored due to age-related differences in drug metabolism. Electroconvulsive therapy may also be an effective treatment course if medications prove ineffective.

Treatment plans for depressed older people must be multifaceted and include family members. Suicide is a major complication of depression in the elderly. The effects of age on suicide rates have been widely studied; in almost all societies, suicide increases as a function of age (Durkheim, 1951). The reports of incidence vary, but generally the elderly make up only 11 percent of the population and account for 25 percent of all reported suicides (Resnick & Cantor, 1970). There are suspicions about the reliability of this figure due to possible underreporting as a result of family embarrassment or attributing death in old age to accident when in reality death was a result of suicide.

Explanations for the high suicide rate in the elderly include the high frequency of widowhood, which is associated with suicide (Bock & Webber, 1972; MacMahon & Pugh, 1965). Resnick and Cantor (1970) suggest that elderly suicide is related to physical and mental traumas. Others propose a correlation between suicide and chronic alcoholism and between suicide and cognitive impairments. The clinician must stay sensitive to the potential for suicide in the recently widowed, recently retired, physically impaired, cognitively impaired, and emotionally disturbed. Suicidal thoughts should be explored in all evaluations of depression in the elderly. The features of ambivalence and suicide attempts or gestures for attention may be less apparent among the elderly who are contemplating suicide. The potential for suicidal behavior as escape from painful reality must be assessed. Depressions and suicidal behaviors among the elderly are treatable with sensitive and timely interventions.

Anxiety

Anxiety is a common psychiatric complaint, and the elderly appear to be as subject to distress from anxiety as other age groups. Clear age patterns, however, are not available. Psychological signs of anxiety include a wide range from worry, apprehension, and anticipation to fear, panic, and terror in the extreme form. Physiological evidence of anxiety involves many systems and can include stomach upset, change in bowel habits, increased heart rate, headaches, and increased muscle tension. Anxiety is often a multifaceted problem; it is sometimes difficult to differentiate from physical diseases such as thyroid disease, tremors, and the silent diseases associated with aging such as painless myocardial infarction, afebrile pneumonia, or appendicitis with abdominal discomfort.

Anxiety is also associated with psychosocial problems common in late life. Cognitive impairments are often accompanied by a variety of anxiety symptoms. In this case, anxiety is a reaction to perceived change, loss, and dysfunction. The relationship of anxiety to alcoholism is complex. Older people may treat anxiety by self-medicating with alcohol, and alcohol can create central nervous system irritability that looks like anxiety, thus creating a vicious cycle.

Attempts have been made to relate physiological changes in arousal, which accompany aging (Eisdorfer, Nowlin, & Wilkie, 1970), to anxiety. However, cause and effect relationships are not clear; increased arousal may be a result, a cause, or a condition associated with anxiety. Attempts to relate central nervous system neurotransmitter changes to anxiety are equally complex.

Common diagnostic categories with major symptoms of anxiety include the neurosis and adjustment disorders. Anxiety neurosis usually has a midlife onset, but due to psychiatric accessibility and avoidance of outreach to the elderly, it may present initially in late life with a lifelong history of psychological distress. The obsessive-compulsive anxiety patterns can also occur in later life with predominant features of perfectionism, isolation of emotional expression, and substitution of ritualistic, repetitive behaviors. Anxiety is a common feature of developmental adjustments, adjustments to change, and adjustments to loss.

Treatment of anxiety in the elderly must be directed by comprehensive assessment and accurate diagnosis. The true nature of psychological discomfort and physical symptoms must be explored. Physical diseases mimicking anxiety as well as the physical diseases associated with anxiety must be treated. Individual and group psychotherapies are useful to enhance the anxious individual's understanding of symptoms, stresses, and adaptations. Stress management and biofeedback techniques with minor adjustments to increase interest and compliance in late life are effective.

The use of medications is dependent on the nature of the anxiety, onset, and contributing factors. Minor tranquilizers are generally viewed as effective short-term treatments when combined with other psychological supports and environmental adjustments. However, use of medications that have potentially sedative, muscle relaxation, and addictive potential must be used with caution. Anxiety should be controlled without oversedation, mild confusional states, impairment in ambulation, gait instability, or support of a drug abuse pattern. Other important aspects of treatment include reengagement or reconnection to the social milieu and review of potential family conflicts that may aggravate anxiety or result from anxiety.

Paranoia

Paranoia is one of the most socially disruptive psychiatric disorders of late life. Symptoms range from mild querulousness, which may be socially irritating, to a personal unrealistic sense of impending threat to a profound and disabling social crisis. Paranoia and suspiciousness present a challenging diagnostic problem as symptoms may outline both a cluster of behaviors and affective and cognitive problems, rather than a unitary behavioral problem (Eisdorfer, 1980). Complete understanding of paranoia in later life requires careful and sensitive review of the intensity of symptoms, the basis of symptoms in reality versus nonreality, and the resulting impact on functional capacities for daily living.

The intensity of symptoms may be usefully viewed along the following continuum: a demanding nature, mild querulousness, social irritation, obvious troublesomeness, and suspiciousness. Suspiciousness is a marker along the continuum of social connection. Sparacino (1978) has pointed out how interpersonal losses of the elderly lead to an impaired use of social consensus and a defense of unrealistically attributing causes for loss to the environment. It is necessary to assess how the individual evaluates environmental information in light of perceptual losses as well. Cooper, Garside, and Kay (1976) studied the role of deafness in paranoia and found that an early-life onset of deafness contributes to development of paranoia later in life. The social impact of deafness can be observed in conversations with older people who may misinterpret, fill in communication gaps by imagining rather than asking for repetition, and generally need to invest more energy in the process of social consensus and reality checking.

Suspiciousness then may be mild, reality-based responses to biopsychosocial stresses or part of the continuum of increasing intensity of paranoia. The more serious end of the continuum includes the following: disabling thought patterns, aggressive arguments, feelings of persecution, intense isolated delusions, delusions of invasion of person and environment, or constant sense of threat to existence. Disorders in this degree of the continuum are clearly distressing to the individuals and those around them. Diagnostic categories include paranoid states with no associated memory or thought disorganization. Deficits are limited to circumscribed specific delusions such as a belief that the upstairs neighbor is playing loud music to annoy or that some vague force is sending poisonous gases through the window. When these deficits are chronic, the individual may well have made adjustments in how and when to share these unique and unusual beliefs. The other major diagnostic category, which includes paranoid symptoms, is that of late-life schizophrenias associated with disorganization of thought processes in addition to delusions and paranoia. Paranoia is also occasionally associated with cognitive impairments or chronic alcoholism.

The total picture of how paranoia affects function can be understood through the use of the functional assessment instrument of Chapter 3. Very often functional deficits are most apparent in social relationships. Paranoia not only painfully disconnects older people from the environment directly; due to popular misunderstanding about the perceived harmfulness of paranoid people, society maintains their disconnection.

Treatment of paranoia must be multifaceted and may include trials of antipsychotic medications (in the severe cases), resocialization, and reconnection to meaningful behavior patterns. When cognitive impairments or perceptual deficits are contributory, they should be completely evaluated and treated. Memory habilitation is helpful in providing a greater sense of control over information. Hearing aids provide greater ease in attaining social consensus and avoiding sensory deprivation. The challenge of paranoia is to integrate these approaches and maintain compliance and cooperation in the disruptive distressed individual. A family-based approach to management of paranoia is presented in Chapter 4.

Psychiatric disorders of depression, anxiety, and paranoia are often treated quietly in the nursing home and institutional environments. All older people, regardless of place of residence, level of function, or age deserve timely and complete evaluations of psychiatric disorders and comprehensive and appropriate treatments.

ALCOHOL AND POLYDRUG ABUSE

Drug abuse and medication misuse among the elderly are generally recognized problems. Statistics for general patterns of drug abuse have not been clearly identified due to a lack of a standard definition of abuse as well as the hidden nature of the problem.

It is well recognized that persons aged 55 and older are the largest consumers of prescribed drugs (Pascarelli & Fisher, 1974). While the majority of these prescriptions are warranted (Geriscope, 1972), there is a professional mandate to evaluate and monitor potential patterns of abuse among the elderly carefully. Inadvertent abuse or misuse of prescribed medication may occur with confusion about the dosage schedule and a tendency to share drugs or hoard medication (Raskind & Eisdorfer, 1976). The combination of prescribed drugs with over-the-counter drugs or alcohol or a general lack of information about the interactive effects of a medication poses a particular problem. Additional drug-related problems among the elderly include excessive self-medication, increased risk of drug interactions, and an increased sensitivity of side effects of medications.

The elderly represent the largest regular users of sedatives, hypnotics, and major and minor tranquilizers (Task Force on Prescription Drugs, 1968). The most frequently abused drugs include the minor tranquilizers, especially the benzodiazopines, and the sedative hypnotics, especially barbiturates (Subby, 1975). Clinical experience suggests that many of those using psychotropic drugs feel that they could not perform their activities of daily living without these agents. These statistics point to a major issue in geriatric health care, questioning the high-frequency use of abusable, prescribed medications within this population. While there is an increasing popular awareness as to the harmful effects of abusive patterns, including prescribed drugs, it is the clinician's responsibility to continue educational efforts and monitor closely the indications and effectiveness of major and minor tranquilizer treatment regimens including the treatment of chronic insomnia with longer-term sedative, hypnotic use.

Other medications have been implicated in abuse patterns, especially among the older population. These include laxatives (Cummings, Sladen, & James, 1974) and aspirin compounds (Morrant, 1975) as well as over-the-counter medications, including sleeping medications, antihistamines, and anticholinergics such as scopolamine, which are found in most over-the-counter nerve medications (Schuckit, 1977).

Identification of drug abuse problems centers around behavior observation of the functioning older person and sensitivity to mild confusional states, imbalance or unsteady gait, slurred speech, frequent falls, a general daze or lethargy, or a distinct difference in alertness and cognitive style.

As in the area of alcohol abuse, there may be an association of loss, feelings of uselessness, age-related stress, or predispositions to use of tranquilizers and sedatives. However, there is no direct evidence that these psychosocial factors have contributed to substance abuse patterns among the aged (Schuckit, 1977).

Treatment of drug abuse begins with an admission of the problem, surrender to withdrawal, and treatment to redo abuse patterns. Education with regard to harmful effects of drug abuse or misuse, social reengagement, and reconnection to the family are recommended modes of treatment. Supportive community services are also an integral part of returning an older person to a drug-free life style.

Identification of Alcoholism

Identification and appropriate treatment of the high percentage of older alcoholics are immediate concerns. In general, all alcoholics underutilize resources of mental health or alcoholism services and deny abuse problems. On a personal level, the older alcohol abuser may suffer shame, anxiety, and remorse in relationship to an alcohol abuse pattern, due to the predominant cultural posture toward such abuse. Our culture continues to define alcoholism popularly at the level of the skid row bum. The older population is personally at risk to continue identification of an alcohol abuse problem at this level only. Families of the older alcoholic also maintain the denial of alcohol abuse problems; the issue remains hidden in the family's closet of skeletons. When the issue of alcohol abuse in the older population is more directly discussed, a long social and cultural tradition of alcohol use as an individual's free choice emerges. The older abuser readily uses this rationalization to defend abusive patterns. The older alcoholic invokes a negative image of aging with concomitant losses of control and rationalizes that alcohol is the only positive recreation available. Another more aggressive but common rationalization points out that one's life is one's own, that drinking is by free choice, or that he or she doesn't have long to live anyway. Family members tend to underreact, supporting these rationalizations, by humoring their older members who drink, or disengaging the older member because of the discomfort with observing destructive alcohol abuse patterns.

Research on the identification of characteristics of older alcoholics is complicated by the family's attitude, demographic variables in a transient or hidden population, significant individual differences, and the ever-present longitudinal research difficulties. The standard method for identification of alcoholism involves identification of problems in family, social, work, and legal areas. In a large study of American drinking behavior by Cahalan, Cisin, and Crossley (1969), there were few areas of difference between younger and older alcoholics. Their study did reveal that older men more often report binge drinking patterns, problems with family, financial problems related to drinking, and legal problems as well as slightly more health problems than younger men. Younger men, on the other hand, reported more symptomatic behavior and psychological dependence on alcohol, including more belligerence and more alcohol-related job problems. These minor differences present a major gap in identification of the older alcoholic who may be retired and not subject to the scrutiny of an employer or an employee assistance program.

Some clinicians argue that alienation from family and years of denial in distancing from the older problem drinker associated with the older alcoholic's lack of mainstream employment and socialization patterns leave them at lower risk to be identified and targeted as problem drinkers. This clinical impression is supported by a study in the Baltimore area (Rathbone-McCuan, Lohn, Levenson, & Hsu, 1976) in which problem drinkers were compared with normal social-drinking age peers. The following differences were noted. The health status for the older drinkers was poorer, with a great number of physical problems. The older problem drinkers appeared to be more alienated from society and peers than elderly normal drinkers; older drinkers reported minimal social participation and minimal sharing of personal life experiences with significant others, including family, friends, and relatives.

In summary, few distinctive differences separate the older alcoholic from the younger alcoholic. Consequently, methods of identification of abuse must be flexible. However, there appear to be three useful definitions or groupings for the patterns of older alcoholism. These definitions relate to age at the onset of the alcoholic drinking pattern. The first group includes "survivors" of a lifelong unremitting pattern of habitual drinking. Glatt and Rosin (1964) suggest that this group is more characteristically identified by their social pathology. The group of lifelong alcoholics is differentiated from a second group, loosely defined as *reactive drinkers*. Psychopathology is more characteristic of this group. Reactive drinkers are further divided into two groups. One group of intermittent reactive drinkers has a history of episodic, recurrent binge drinking, which may be aggravated by the stresses and loneliness of aging. Life histories reveal an earlier life-escape pattern of drinking and problem solving through heavy alcohol abuse. The other type of reactive drinkers, the third group, is more clearly identified by recent onset. These recent reactive problem drinkers exhibit a lifelong history of adequate coping and vocational and social achievement with abuses a fairly recent life event. Recent history includes stresses resulting in irritability and social withdrawal, and significant stressors such as retirement or loss of spouse as precipitants of heavy drinking. Bailey, Haberman, and Alksne (1965) point out that elderly widows are at highest risk to develop this type of reactive drinking. The relative proportion of elderly alcoholics who could be identified as survivors, intermittent, reactive, or recent onset drinkers is unclear at this time. Furthermore, classification of alcohol abuse according to the amount of abuse does not change the treatment goal of sobriety, but it does provide a framework for initial identification.

Historical Context of Specific Concerns for Alcoholism

A long sociocultural history enforces freedom of choice of consumption of alcoholic beverages. The current generation of people over 65 have lived through the period of the Volstead Act, which prohibited alcoholic beverages. They approached young adulthood just as prohibition was repealed and the entire country was embroiled in emotional conflict over the subject. Further, they may have difficulty identifying alcohol as an abusable drug when alcohol has been integrated into their lives and culture. For them, abuse may be defined by the image of the younger generation smoking pot or using LSD, heroin, and cocaine.

Professional Response

There is a well-recognized professional avoidance of treating the elderly in general and the elderly alcoholic in particular. Alcoholism treatment centers challenge the motivation of all potential patients prior to admission. The recidivism rate of the surviving older drinker is high. Programs are generally designed for young adults to the middle-aged living in the cultural mainstream, still part of the work force. Treatment centers often have a callous approach to treatment failures and "therapeutically discharge" older people who are unsuccessful in the programs. Marden (1976) points out that a differential criterion for acceptance in treatment exists for older alcoholics as agencies prefer to concentrate services and resources on patients who can demonstrate "success."

Differential Diagnosis

Alcoholism does not represent a difficult diagnostic challenge. Alcohol is a problem when it disrupts family life, social relationships and work, including volunteer work or retirement activities, and creates legal problems such as public intoxication or driving while intoxicated. Accurate diagnosis requires an a number of related diagnostic issues of extreme importance. The effects of alcoholism may result in physical deterioration, gait instability with frequent falls, malnutrition, and dementias. Clinicians must then systematically explore these conditions and determine those directly related to long-term alcohol abuse and those possibly related to other chronic diseases.

There are a number of interrelationships between neurological and psychiatric disorders caused by alcoholism (Bennett, 1977). Acute brain syndromes are associated with the withdrawal syndrome of tremulousness, sleep disturbance, muscle aches, agitation, nausea, anxiety, and depression. Impending delirium tremens includes shakiness, sweating, and low-grade fever related to the decreasing concentration of alcohol within the central nervous system. Other manifestations of alcohol withdrawal may include alcohol hallucinosis with auditory, accusatory, and persecutory hallucinations. Delirium tremens represents full-blown manifestations of alcohol withdrawal characterized by visual and auditory hallucinations, confusion, disorientation, gross and irregular tremor, possible high fever, tachycardia, increased blood pressure, and seizures. Delirium tremens is life threatening to the aged alcoholic, with hyperthermia or peripheral vascular collapse the usual cause of death (Cohen, 1976).

The chronic brain syndromes associated with alcoholic deterioration and various stages of advanced brain disease include Wernicke-Korsakoff psychosis and alcoholic deterioration. Stages of intermittent deterioration from a clinical definition include sociopathic behavior, emotional lability, amnesic episodes, and an exaggeration of preexisting personality styles (Bennett, Mowery, & Fort, 1960). Personality changes manifested in the intermittent stage of alcoholic brain disease include hostility, poor judgment, emotional lability, absence of insight, pathological lying, and rationalization of drinking. Biological responses include memory blackouts, delirium, or recurrent seizures in addition to the acute withdrawal reactions. The Wernicke-Korsakoff syndrome is also associated with evidence of severe vitamin B deficiency. In its full-blown state, it is not reversible and appears after a long history of drinking associated with malnutrition and the vitamin deficiency. Variable memory deficits, confabulation, and emotional lability are also present. The essential features of Korsakoff psychosis include a retrograde amnesia and anteriorgrade amnesia. Ocular palsies may be present and indicate the Wernicke syndrome.

Etiology

Various authors have presented hypotheses for the etiology of alcoholism. Pascarelli and Fisher (1974) hypothesized reactions to alienation, poverty, and feelings of low status and lack of valuing by society. Bergman and Amir (1973) interview, medical record review, and collateral interviews. However, there are hypothesized feelings of uselessness and dependency. These conditions may be associated; however, there is no clear evidence that they contribute directly to alcoholism. The effect of retirement on the rate of alcoholism is unclear.

Data from Cahalan, Cisin, and Crossley (1969) point to a clear drop in the percentage of heavy drinking and a rise in abstinence or infrequent drinking at age 65. One explanation of this phenomenon suggests the differential that the increased mortality rate for heavy drinkers indeed results in a lower life expectancy (Schmidt & de Lint, 1969) and readjusts the percentages at this age. Drew (1968) favors a view of alcoholism as a "self limiting disease" with evidence of spontaneous remission explaining the change in percentages at age 65. A sociological explanation for the drop in heavy drinking among men of 24 percent from age 60 to 64 to 7 percent at age 65 and above suggests that heavy drinking is associated with job stresses and frustration where drinking is socially facilitated on the job (Gomberg, 1980). Likewise, there is a drop in the proportion of women who drink heavily with the major drop occurring at age 50, earlier than for men. It has been hypothesized that this relates to a change in sex role behavior for women and greater self-expression and acceptance (Neugarten & Gutmann, 1968).

Longitudinal studies considering the genetic predisposition for alcoholism among older people are not available. Statistical evidence of the magnitude of the problem of alcoholism among the elderly is complicated by the fact that available service facilities use different sample populations and definitions of alcohol abuse. The most widely accepted statistic available suggests that 2 to 10 percent of individuals over age 60 and residing in the community suffer from alcoholism (Schuckit & Pastor, 1978). When considering populations in nursing home settings and hospital-based populations, the reported prevalence rates range from 25 percent (Reading, 1974) to 45 percent (Gomberg, 1977).

Current Treatment Modalities

Clinicians have debated the special treatment needs of the elderly as a unique population in alcohol treatment. Intervention and referral for treatment may be more difficult due to the individual's attitudes, prejudices, and social and vocational disengagement as well as the family's denial, alienation, and long history of avoidance of the subject. However, once older alcoholics are admitted to treatment, the prognosis is often better for the elderly than for the middle-aged (Zimberg, 1974; Pascarelli, 1974); special treatment needs disappear. Schuckit (1977) reports that 73 percent of alcoholics over the age of 60 complete treatment compared to 40 percent of younger alcoholics. Poor prognosis is more evident for alcoholic populations with associated brain deterioration than for the older alcoholic whose drinking is a reaction to loss and stress.

While basic treatment needs of the older alcoholic are not unique, reconnecting them to a larger social network is vital. Family therapy for elderly problem drinkers is relatively new though it is recognized (Gomberg, 1975). Rathbone-McCuan and Triegaardt (1978) have emphasized a family approach including the multigenerational family system. Increasing the family's understanding of abuse patterns, defense mechanisms, treatment possibilities, and prognosis does a great deal to reconnect the older drinker.

Acute withdrawal of the elderly is managed in the usual way, with specific attention to vitamin replacement and control of initial withdrawal symptoms with drug therapy for sedation once the delirium has cleared, with gradual reduction within the first week. Good nutrition should be maintained, and fluids should be encouraged in order to restore electrolyte balance. Associated deficiencies in magnesium are treated with parenteral magnesium when evident. Multivitamin therapy, especially B-complex, is equally important. Treatment of any associated chronic disease is also important in this population, who may have ignored good, ongoing medical attention.

Other specifics of treatment include attention to nursing cares demanded by the complexity of associated physical problems. Occasionally, deficits in vision and hearing interfere with the didactic parts of treatment programs and must be compensated by use of larger print reading material and auditory presentation of materials through tapes or readings. Memory delays and cognitive failures associated with alcoholic brain deterioration also have the potential to interfere. Memory habilitation efforts, external memory storage, and environmental compensation should be provided to facilitate acquisition of treatment information.

The long-range treatment planning for alcohol abuse among older people should include follow-up to assure successful transition to community settings and reestablishment of a social network through outpatient Alcoholics Anonymous (AA) or attendance at senior citizens centers or church groups, for instance. Social services are useful for transportation problems, financial planning, and management. Alcoholism is very likely to go untreated in nursing home environments (Snyder, 1977). Patterns of alcohol overuse in nursing home populations should be identified wherever possible and included in available outpatient treatment programs.

Outreach education to older community members with specific education about the harmful effects of alcohol, dangers of alcohol and polydrug use, and education about the decreased tolerance to alcohol with increasing age are vital. Education about the realistic prognosis is equally vital.

SEXUAL DYSFUNCTION

Sexuality

Sexuality and sexual expression are major concerns in late life. Sexual expression remains a uniquely individual psychological issue throughout the life span with different meanings, purposes, and values. This issue, however, is subject to influences of public attitude, misinformation, and cultural anxiety. Sexuality and sexual expression in late life have only recently been examined objectively. The effect of public attitude and misinformation on the private sexual behaviors of older adults remains unexplored and subject to the individual psychological filters of experience.

Butler and Lewis (1976) outline societal attitudes toward sexuality in late life with the following generally assumed myths: (1) older people do not have sexual desires; (2) older people are unable to perform sexually; (3) older people are physically fragile; (4) they are physically unattractive, therefore undesirable; and (5) sexuality in late life is perverse and shameful. The male in particular suffers from anxieties about impotence with increasing age, in keeping with cultural myths. The aging woman suffers from the general psychological trauma culturally expected in menopause and loss of "sexuality."

Individual attitudes influence sexual expression in later life as well. For older men, especially those with known heart disease, personal fears of death as a result of exertion during the sexual act and subsequent heart attack are widely recognized. Individual uncertainties and lack of information about normal age-related sexual changes also inhibit sexual behaviors.

Research findings in the area of sexuality during later life are incomplete and obscured by the highly personal nature of the subject. However, studies of sexual desire—e.g., Kinsey, Pomeroy, and Martin (1948); Newman and Nichols (1960); and Masters and Johnson (1970)—point out that desire continues well into the final life stage. Newman and Nichols (1960) interviewed subjects aged 60 to 93 and report that 54 percent remained sexually active with no significant decline in interest generally occurring before age 75. The reported decline of interest and decrease in sexuality in 25 percent of the individuals was a result of illness of self or spouse. Evidence suggests that people over the age of 75 who engaged in sexual activity at a young age continue into late life and that a consistent sexual pattern helps to maintain continued sexual expression and satisfaction.

The physical correlations of sexual performance in the normal mature male include a delayed ejaculation and a longer time to achieve an erection; however, neither appears to affect overall performance and satisfaction. Normal age-related changes in the female include vaginal atrophy and decreased lubrication, which may interfere with performance and satisfaction.

Declines in sexual performance for the most part are related to changes in general physical health. Impotence is frequently associated with an increased prevalence of diabetes, the increase in vascular-autonomic insufficiency, the increased prevalence of hypertension, and prostate enlargement, which is accompanied by an increased use of medications that potentially have impotence as a side effect. Surgical procedures for the treatment of prostatic hypertrophy have been known to cause a decrease or loss of potency in 5 to 40 percent (Madorsky, Ashamalla, Schussler, Lyons, & Miller, 1976) and retrograde ejaculation in 80 to 90 percent of the males studied. Nevertheless, the most common cause of impotence among older men has a psychological basis noted in societal expectation and reinforced by ill health, obesity, and increased sensitivity to alcohol and depression (Comfort, 1980).

Menopause has a variety of effects on the sexual behavior of women because of individual psychological expectations and cultural assumptions. For some women, freedom from reproductive potential brings about an increase in sexual interest. In others, the loss of reproductive potential triggers a sense of loss of femininity. Hysterectomies do not appear to change sexual desire or performance in women; however, mastectomies may affect sexual expression because of psychological side effects.

Lifelong sociosexual roles, perception of cultural expectations, and socially propagated anxieties about sexual expression in later life appear to have the greatest influences on sexual expression of older people. Cameron and Biber (1973) have reported a decrease in fantasies with increasing age. Fantasy is one of the most significant variables in sexual arousal. If fantasizing is reduced, sexual desire may be affected as well.

Treatment of sexual dysfunctions in later life should be initiated with similar vigor and commitment as for other age groups. Masters and Johnson (1970) have found older males responsive to treatment of sexual dysfunction. A higher failure rate is reported, but that may be attributed to the duration of the pathology prior to referral and subsequent delay rather than directly related to treatment issues.

Adequate treatment of sexual dysfunctions of older people requires complete physical and psychological evaluation. Exploration of the psychological aspects should be accomplished in a forthright manner respecting the older individual's perceptions, values, and attitudes. The clinician should provide information about normal male and female age changes and be responsive to any expressed needs for additional information such as discussion of masturbation in the absence of a partner and discussion of sexual tensions.

Supportive therapy should be available to those with long-term problems. Some of the psychological issues warranting attention include performance anxieties, the meaning and value of guilt, feelings about sexuality after the death of the spouse, and concerns about a lack of appropriate sexual partners. Butler and Lewis (1976) point out that the special abilities of older people to develop a second language of sex or a growing capacity to develop new levels of intimacy and communication in a love relationship should be a part of ongoing sexual counseling.

Nursing homes should provide relevant information to residents, establish rules for privacy, and be aware of how staff attitudes influence the sexuality between residents or others. Sexual expression within a nursing home should deserve the same respect and considerations as sexual behavior of the larger community-based population.

BIOPHYSICAL CONCERNS

A balanced presentation of psychological distress in aging must deal with older people's concern with their changing biological capacity. Much of the literature on aging makes a clear point that age itself is not a disease, impairment, disability, or handicap. However, Butler and Lewis (1982) point out that in reality 86 percent of older people have some form of chronic health problem. As a result, they are required to see doctors more frequently, follow special diets and exercises, use medications, participate in rehabilitative treatment, and make additional provisions and more changes in their daily routines. Health problems are a reality that threatens identity, distorts emotional responses, and activates fear and anxiety about death.

Theoretical approaches to changing biological capacities and increasing frequency of health problems with age are wide ranging and in diverse sources. Schaie (1981) states that a complete view of aging must consider (1) normative occurrence of events that are implicit in biological characteristics of aging; (2) normative changes that are culturally programmed to occur at a given life stage; and (3) nonnormative personal accidents or pathologies that appear to be signs of premature aging. In other words, this framework begins to differentiate normative and pathological biologically based change as well as normative nonbiologically based change.

Schaie (1981) summarizes theoretical approaches to age-related biological change from a developmental perspective. The general contours of adult development are illuminated in the three following models. The adult stability model refers to behaviors whose biological constraints remain stable throughout maturity, such as cognitive abilities and personality traits. The model of irreversible decrement is more commonly accepted in discussions of age-related change. The final and possibly most relevant model is that of decrement with compensation. For example, a progressive decrement in hearing may be compensated by use of a hearing aid; visual losses may be compensated by glasses. Changes in behavior may represent a failure of the natural compensatory mechanisms in the face of increasing decrement.

Within the scientific research realm, approaches to changes in biological capacity and illness among the aged are equally varied and as diverse as the psychosocial developmental models. Aging is assumed to be related to a natural decline in functional efficiency of cells, tissues, and organ systems. The general term *degeneration* is diffuse. The changes of the individual organ systems as well as the changes of the interdependency of organ systems remain unique to the individual. Interactions of cellular change, organ system change, and possible change in regulatory or control mechanisms have only recently captured research attention (Shock, 1977). However, the overall effect of decreased biological adaptive capacity is widely accepted.

Older people do not age faster than younger people but have accumulated more gradual loss of function over a greater length of time. Rowe (1981) points out marked variation in rates of age-related loss of function in individual organ systems within the aging individual. He cautions against referring to normal age changes as harmless. For example, "normal" age-related change in carbohydrate intolerance may not be harmless. "Normal" increases in blood pressure with age may have adverse effects despite being considered normative.

A practical clinical approach to health problems and biological change with increased age has recently been summarized by the Federated Council for Internal Medicine (Geriatric Medicine, 1981) describing the following characteristics of older patients. Older patients tend to have (1) multiple and complex diseases; (2) altered functional response of many organ systems; (3) chronic illnesses; (4) greater severity of acute illness with slower recovery; (5) functional impairments limiting independent living; (6) fragile response to illness, interventions, and stress; (7) unstable economic and social supports; and (8) limitations in the reversibility of impairments, with management goals often restricted to maintenance rather than cure.

Besdine (1981) provides another useful clinical approach in a discussion of diseases that are unique to old age or diseases that manifest differently in old age. Examples of diseases that are unique to old age include decubiti (bed sores), ulcers, diabetic hyperosmolar nonketotic coma, stroke, osteoporosis, osteoarthritis, hip fracture, falls, prostatic cancer, chronic lymphatic leukemia, basal cell carcinoma (skin cancer), Parkinson's disease, and dementias, to name a few. He describes a second group of diseases that behave differently and present in unusual ways among older people. These include such diseases as masked thyrotoxicosis, painless myocardial infarction, silent pulmonary embolism, afebrile pneumonia, malignant diseases, myxedema, depression, and drug intoxication.

The rehabilitation medicine model provides still another clinical approach to the biological change associated with aging. Blake (1981) emphasizes an increased need for innovative rehabilitation programs to deal with the increased incidence of disability among older people. Specific types of rehabilitation are necessary for older people who have survived major biological catastrophes such as heart attacks, strokes, and cancer with resulting residual impairments. General types of rehabilitation are necessary for those who have avoided the major disabling diseases but suffer from general declines in biological capacity.

Butler and Lewis (1982) have described a humanistic approach to biological change and physical illness. They point out the older person's feelings of helplessness and vulnerability in the face of illness. Illness challenges a sense of pride and self-reliance as the physical changes interfere with normal daily routines. According to Butler and Lewis, "body monitoring" or an increased attention to routine bodily processes begins in middle age and continues into late life. Attention may be adaptive and preventive in some persons. In others such increased attention to bodily processes leads to obsessive ruminations and somatizing.

From a variety of approaches, biological changes and health problems associated with aging do threaten the evolving identity of the older person. Biological changes interact with psychological distresses in complex ways. Biological changes and health problems aggravate psychological adjustment, and psychological distress aggravates biological change and health problems. Comprehensive discussion of individual health problems and biological changes is beyond the scope of this text. However, some of the major concerns are briefly reviewed from a family perspective of concern and include nutrition and exercise activity patterns.

Nutrition

Complete review of the nutritional needs, requirements, and behaviors of older people leads to a number of major concerns. Clearly, the elderly are at risk to develop nutritional deficiencies, undernutrition, nutritional imbalances, and problems with diseases such as diabetes, hypertension, cardiovascular disease, and osteoporosis, which are all affected by nutritional intake (Todhunter & Darby, 1978).

Assessment of nutritional problems in old age demands review of biological, psychological, and social variables. Biological changes that affect nutrition include dentures and oral cavity diseases, diseases or changes that result in decreased gastric acid or biliary tract or pancreatic disease, acute illnesses including fevers, and cancers that affect appetite. Alcoholism and depression are also well-recognized influences on adequate nutrition. Psychological issues that influence nutrition include boredom, monotony, poor self-esteem, loss of mobility, and loss of food preparation skills. Perceptual changes of decreased vision and hearing may result in avoidance of social gatherings or restaurants due to embarrassment or inability to communicate in large groups and in dimly lit places (Busse, 1978). The elderly notice a troubling loss of satisfaction with taste and smell in high frequency (Cohen & Gitman, 1959). Change in food habits, food resources, and attitudes is significant in the nutritional histories of older people.

Social issues that affect nutrition in the elderly include loneliness, a sense of forsakenness, joblessness, low socioeconomic status, and lack of a social opportunity at mealtimes (Todhunter & Darby, 1978). A social history of older people with nutritional problems often reveals that earlier in life mealtime had been a major social event of the day, a time to share experiences and catch up on social relationships. The severe losses of old age restrict this opportunity.

Nutritional requirements of older people have been studied with one resulting recommended change. Calorie requirements decrease with age due to decreased activity levels, change in the body's metabolism that results in less energy required, and a general decrease in cell mass. The nutrient need for vitamins, minerals, and proteins, however, does not change appreciably. Furthermore, digestive changes may decrease absorption of minerals and vitamins, making them clearly more important in maintaining a balance. The challenge for the older person then is to maintain good nutrient values in food while decreasing calorie intake. The most widely recommended way of doing this involves maintaining good protein sources such as meats, fish, milk, and vegetables (Harper, 1978).

Common nutritional problems that require specific treatments include the nutritional anemias such as iron deficiency and macrocytic anemias of folic acid deficiency or vitamin B12 deficiency. Vitamin C deficiency commonly results from a lack of fresh fruits and vegetables. All these biological, psychological, and social variables contribute to a complex malnutrition picture with avitaminosis and protein deficiency.

A number of diseases are influenced by nutrition. Adult-onset diabetes mellitus can often be controlled by diet alone when carbohydrate calories are restricted. Cardiovascular problems associated with hyperlipedemia and hypertension require control of saturated fats and sodium intake. Calcium supplementation in osteoporosis is not proven to be curative but is indicated to provide maximum dietary protection against progress of the disease (Todhunter & Darby, 1978).

Further research in nutrition and disease processes in general promises to answer important questions related to aging and nutrition. Such questions include the effect of dietary fat on atherosclerosis, the effect of salt on hypertension, the effect of fiber on metabolism, and the effect of a wide range of proposed carcinogens on development of cancers.

Exercise

Physiological changes that accompany age do not seriously limit an older person's potential for exercise. In fact, exercise is generally accepted as an effective means of slowing the rate of age-related decline. Decline in biological functions may be directly related to a person's exercise history. Older people, however, need a more individualized exercise program.

Research findings on the effects of exercise on aging and different aspects of functioning are unclear. There is a noticeable lack of research focus on exercise and older people. Existing studies are difficult to interpret because results of young-old companions are made on subjects who are actually middle-aged and not old. Biological effects of exercise on psychosocial variables similarly lack meaningful comparisons. DeVries and Adams (1972) report that acute exercise of low intensity effectively reduced muscle tension in older people. Diesfeldt and Diesfeldt-Groenendyk (1977) report that exercise significantly improves memory function in a cognitively impaired apathetic older population. Other studies offer contradictory results, and the impact of social effects of an exercise group from the biophysical effects are unclear.

Nevertheless, daily exercise should be a part of routine physical care of older people at home and in institutions. Exercise programs can be individualized according to a person's capacity and designed for sitting, standing, wheelchair-bound, or bedridden older people. Important psychological issues include the possible initial resistance to exercise because of negative attitudes. Psychological benefits include an increased sense of body control and confidence. Social benefits may well include increased positive contact through group exercise programs. Many lifelong interests, routines, and social activities include a fair amount of exercise and should be continued into old age whenever possible. Examples include dancing, gardening, sports, walking to get the mail, or walking to social activities or church.

FAMILY CONCERNS: ELDER ABUSE

Elder abuse and neglect represent a dramatic form of intergenerational conflict. Elder abuse has only recently come to the attention of professionals and researchers, and consequently is poorly understood in its entirety. However, existing research shows a consistent pattern of abuse of a physically or mentally impaired elderly person by a family member.

Many factors help to keep elder abuse hidden within the family. Unfortunately, ageism attitudes and stereotypes may perpetuate neglect and harsh treatments of older people "because they're too old and senile to know the difference." When society lacks an accepted role for older people, denial of their rights lays a foundation for abuse. The elderly become easy victims as the stereotypes of disengaged and nonassertive older individuals.

In addition to ageism and stereotypes, lack of community awareness of the issue of elder abuse further operates to keep it hidden. The frightening reality of community indifference and misinterpretation of observed/suspected abuse as a private family matter exists. Few known intervention programs exist, and the process for seeking help remains unclear for the abused as well as the abuser.

Victims or abusers rarely seek outside help specifically for abuse. In fact, one study in Massachusetts (O'Rourke, 1981) found that in at least 70 percent of abuse cases cited, active involvement of a community member outside the abuse situation was required before the abuse came to the attention of professionals.

The community and professionals may be protecting themselves from this emotionally loaded issue by the defense of denial. The models of child abuse and spouse abuse point to the practical reality of the tremendous emotional load surrounding identification and intervention in abuse cases. The practical reality of elder abuse is no different. Emotions range from complete disbelief to surprise to rage because of the injustices, inequities, and reality of the suffering.

As outsiders to the abuse situation, professionals new to the field may find that empathy and objectivity are difficult to maintain in the face of major suffering. Professionals must simultaneously integrate feelings of repulsion, depression, or fear with patience and commitment to changing family patterns.

Difficulties in documenting abuse represent another major factor keeping it hidden from view. Few states have mandatory reporting laws; consequently, a formalized standardized reporting method has not been developed. Alleged or real cognitive impairments of the abused elder complicate initial documentation of the abuse. In cases of financial abuse, banking accounts of the elder may have been established as conjoint with the family member, making documentation of abuse extremely difficult for an outsider.

The greatest factor keeping elder abuse a hidden issue may well be the resistance of the abused individual. This resistance has been attributed to a fear of retaliation by the abuser, including complete rejection of care, escalated abuse, placement outside the family setting, or withheld portions of the current level of care. In addition, feelings of kinship and love make it difficult for the abused elder to admit family abuse patterns without a personal sense of shame.

The abused victim may also resign himself or herself to the fact of abuse or simply refuse outside help. Individual resistance to acknowledge abuse creates a legal dilemma concerning the rights of privacy and self-determination of the abused as well as ethical dilemmas concerning the abused person's right to refuse professional intervention. The question of competency can be raised when an abused elder chooses to stay in an abusive situation without outside help. However, the authority to intervene in this way is limited, and competency laws are often vague.

There is clearly a lack of definitive research into the issues of elder abuse. The research that does exist suffers from a lack of a common classification system for the various types of abuse. Lack of a standardized methodology and sampling makes comparisons and integration of existing research data difficult. Lack of a current data base creates a need for highly individualized professional management along every step of the way.

Definitions of Abuse

A basic review of current definitions of abuse outlines part of the complexity. The Massachusetts study (O'Rourke, 1981) defined abuse as "the willful infliction of physical pain, injury or debilitating mental anguish, unreasonable confinement or deprivation by a caretaker of services which are necessary to maintain mental and physical health" (p. 7). This definition outlines the basic forms of abuse apparent in other research in Maryland, Michigan, and Ohio (O'Rourke, 1981):

- *physical abuse,* including physical assault as well as sexual assault
- *psychological abuse,* including verbal assault and threats, provoking fear and isolation
- *basic neglect* of human needs of food, clothing, companionship, medical attention and treatment, and assistance with personal cares
- *material abuse,* including theft or misuse of money, property, or belongings

Material abuse can be expanded to include financial abuses of embezzlement, improper charges, and consumer fraud. Institutional abuse is also recognized as a form of abuse and includes overutilization of medications, failure to secure adequate medical attention, excessive use of restraints, and inadequate attention to restoration of functional skills.

Intervention in elder abuse requires a clear understanding of the forces and dynamics involved. However, review of available literature reveals that no single dynamic explains elder abuse. Cases must be handled in individualized ways. A number of issues in regard to dynamics emerge from differing theoretical and research perspectives. Straus, Gelles, and Steinmetz (1980) reviewed social causes of family violence, pointing out a changing norm of American society that supports and legitimizes the use of violence to solve problems, punish, educate, and control. According to their studies, violent behavior is learned within the family context and becomes transgenerational, especially in conjunction with stress. While their work does not include elder abuse specifically, this theoretical framework can be applied to a family's caregiving to the elderly. The problems of the elderly are complex behaviorally, psychologically, and physically. Use of violence to control problems of the elderly is not an illogical extrapolation. It seems unlikely that transgenerational patterns of violence would stop at midlife (Block & Sinnott, 1979).

Failure to resolve the filial crisis (Blenkner, 1965) may contribute to elder abuse. The developmental task of the adult child involves overcoming adolescent rebelliousness and emancipation issues to view adult parents beyond the parental role. Potentially many family conflicts could surface in the form of bickering, arguing, and abusing. In addition, Block and Sinnott (1979) point out that adult children may not anticipate caregiving to parents after responsibilities of child rearing have ceased and may well view caregiving to elders as stressful.

All of these considerations are vitally important in elder abuse interventions. Interventions of necessity must be system-oriented in order to determine the nature of forces operating in the environment of older people. Interventions must not jeopardize the security of the abused individual. The goal of resolving family stress and reconciling family conflicts may be reasonable, and initial interventions must be aware of forces that alienate abusive families. If permanent separation of abuser from abused is necessary, supportive help or referrals should be offered to all family members.

SUMMARY

Despite a high risk for psychiatric illness, the elderly comprise only 2 to 4 percent of the cases in outpatient clinics (Eisdorfer & Stotsky, 1977). This disparity has not been systematically explored through research methods. However, there are a number of important clinical interpretations of the resistance to initial intervention for psychiatric distress among the elderly.

The most obvious source of resistance to psychiatric intervention may lie with the older person's misperception of the true nature of the psychiatric diagnostic process and intervention. The current older population has lived through a time of major change in psychiatric services and may have had experiences at earlier times in their lives with "insane asylums," poor farms, and exposure to a more primitive psychiatric intervention that continues to have a high emotional charge.

The younger population generally has benefited from a greater exposure to psychological jargon and therapy processes. There have been few widespread mental health education attempts directed specifically for the elderly population. The older individual may harbor the unchallenged belief that psychological distresses are part of growing older rather than part of a treatable illness. If the older person does admit to feelings of psychological distress, it may be an affront to his or her pride to seek help from outside psychological resources to compensate. Further, he or she may choose initially to seek out support during times of distress from clergy, family members, and psychologically oriented and supportive neighbors. Individual resistance to psychiatric intervention may also be based on a lack of appreciation for the full range of current outpatient or day services and the expectation that care is limited to institutions and hospitals.

The older individual's family may also resist psychiatric intervention due to misinformation about the process and potential outcome. They, too, may attribute the psychological distress to the aging process and passively resign themselves to disordered behavior, psychological symptoms, and change in function. The individual and family may tend to view psychiatric symptoms as related to physical change or illness that historically has been the realm of the primary care physician. Long-term relationships with primary care physicians may increasingly become an important support for initial identification of psychological distress and subsequent psychiatric referral.

The primary care physician, however, is also subject to a number of resistances as well. Lack of attention to the subtleties of psychological distress, minimization of the psychological symptoms, or attribution of psychological change to part of the aging process may be weighed against the time-consuming task of a psychiatric referral. While the general medical community has an increasing appreciation for the skills and abilities of psychiatrists, attitudes toward the aged continue to influence the referral process. It is not uncommon in the 1980s to hear a primary care physician say that "she's too old for psychiatric care to be of any value." The primary physician may fear lack of family cooperation in the process or may not develop a working relationship with a psychiatrist especially interested and trained in working with elderly people.

It is necessary at any level of referral to pay particular attention to the initial facilitation of psychiatric evaluation and the varieties of resistances. The nature of the psychiatric evaluation process may not result in an immediate concrete product or result that is evident to the older person. Consequently, it is also necessary for referring sources to help maintain and reinforce a commitment to complete psychiatric evaluation given the presentation of psychiatric symptoms. This process has on occasion been complicated by the primary physician's attitudes and the skill level of psychiatry in general, as well as the product of a psychiatric evaluation. Psychiatric diagnosis and recommendations are not as concrete as a laboratory test result of hemoglobin count, and there may be misunderstandings. The process of psychiatric intervention in the elderly is more typically described as one of ongoing problem solving, reevaluation, and treatment readjustment.

A number of studies have also outlined the psychiatrist's general resistance to working with the elderly (Arnhoff & Kumbar, 1970). The lack of interest, training, and services definitely influences the psychiatric intervention process.

Finally, the elderly themselves may view psychiatric services as a luxury. Adjusted-fee or free community outpatient clinics may be viewed as charity and rejected as well.

The complexity and frequency of psychological distress among the aged, combined with their resistance to complete evaluation and the shortage of service providers, create a true challenge when approaching specific concerns.

REFERENCES

Arnhoff, F., & Kumbar, A. *The nation's psychiatrists: 1970 survey.* Washington, D.C.: American Psychological Association, 1970.

Bailey, M.B., Haberman, P.W., & Alksne, H. The epidemiology of alcoholism in an urban residential area. *Quarterly Journal of Studies on Alcohol,* 1965, *26,* 19–40.

Baltes, P.B., & Schaie, K.W. Aging and IQ: The myths of the twilight years. *Psychology Today,* March 1974, pp. 35–40.

Ban, T.A. The treatment of depressed geriatric patients. *American Journal of Psychotherapy,* 1978, *32,* 93–95.

Bennett, A.E. *Alcoholism and the brain.* New York: Stratton Intercontinental Medical Book Corp., 1977.

Bennett, A.E., Mowery, G.L., & Fort, J.T. Brain damage from chronic alcoholism: The diagnosis of intermediate stage of alcoholic brain disease. *American Journal of Psychiatry,* 1960, *116,* 705–711.

Bergman, S., & Amir, M. Crime and delinquency among the aged in Israel. *Geriatrics,* 1973, *28,* 149–157.

Besdine, R.W. The content of geriatric medicine. In A. Somers & D. Fabian (Eds.), *The geriatric imperative: An introduction to gerontology and clinical geriatrics.* New York: Appleton-Century-Crofts, 1981.

Blake, R. Disabled older persons: A demographic analysis. *Journal of Rehabilitation,* October/November/December 1981, pp. 19–27.

Blenkner, M. Social work and family relationships in later life, with some thoughts on filial maturity. In E. Shanas & F.G. Streib (Eds.), *Social structure and the family: Generational relations.* Englewood Cliffs, N.J.: Prentice-Hall, 1965.

Block, M.R., & Sinnott, J.D. (Eds.). *The battered elder syndrome.* College Park: University of Maryland Center on Aging, 1979.

Bock, E.W., & Webber, I.L. Suicide among the elderly: Isolating widowhood and mitigating alternatives. *Journal of Marriage and the Family,* 1972, *15,* 24–30.

Botwinick, J. *Cognitive process in maturity and old age.* New York: Springer, 1967.

Brody, E.M. *Long-term care: A practical guide.* New York: Human Sciences Press, 1977.

Brody, E.M., Kleban, M.H., Lawton, M.P., & Silverman, H. Excess disabilities of mentally impaired aged: Impact of individualized treatment. *Gerontologist,* 1971, *11,* 124–133.

Burke, D.M., & Light, L.L. Memory and aging: The role of retrieval processes. *Psychological Bulletin,* 1981, *90* (3), 513–546.

Busse, E.W. How mind, body and environment influence nutrition in the elderly. *Postgraduate Medicine,* 1978, *63,* 118–125.

Butler, R.N. Toward a psychiatry of the life cycle: Implications of socio-psychological studies of the aging process for policy and practice of psychotherapy. In A. Simon & L. Epstein (Eds.), *Aging and modern society: Psychosocial and medical aspects.* Washington, D.C.: American Psychological Association, 1968.

Butler, R.N. Psychiatry and the elderly: An overview. *American Journal of Psychiatry,* 1975a, *132* (9), 893–900.

Butler, R.N. *Why survive? Being old in America.* New York: Harper and Row, 1975b.

Butler, R.N., & Lewis, M.I. *Sex after sixty: A guide for men and women for their later years.* New York: Harper and Row, 1976.

Butler, R.N., & Lewis, M.I. *Aging and mental health: Positive psychosocial and biomedical approaches.* St. Louis: C.V. Mosby, 1982.

Cahalan, D., Cisin, I.H., & Crossley, H.M. *American drinking practices.* New Brunswick, N.J.: Rutgers University Press, 1969.

Cameron, P., & Biber, H. Sexual thoughts throughout the life span. *Gerontologist,* 1973, *13,* 144-147.

Cohen, S. Alcohol withdrawal syndromes. *Drug Abuse and Alcoholism Newsletter,* 1976, *5* (5), 1-3.

Cohen, T., & Gitman, L. Oral complaints and taste perception in the aged. *Journal of Gerontology,* 1959, *14,* 294-298.

Comfort, A. Sexuality in later life. In J.E. Birren & R.B. Sloan (Eds.), *Handbook of mental health and aging.* Englewood Cliffs, N.J.: Prentice-Hall, 1980.

Constantinidis, J. Is Alzheimer's disease a major form of senile dementia? Clinical, anatomical and genetic data. In R. Katzman, R. Terry, & K. Bick (Eds.), *Alzheimer's disease: Senile dementia and related disorders.* New York: Raven Press, 1978.

Cooper, A.F., Garside, R.F., & Kay, D.W. A comparison of deaf and non-deaf patients with an affective psychosis. *British Journal of Psychiatry,* 1976, *129,* 532-538.

Crook, T., & Gershon, S. *Strategies for the development of an effective treatment for senile dementia.* New Canaan, Conn.: Mark Powley Associates, 1981.

Cummings, J.H., Sladen, G.E., & James, O.F.W. Laxative-induced diarrhea: A continuing clinical problem. *British Medical Journal,* 1974, *1,* 537-541.

Davies, P. Studies on the neurochemistry of central cholinergic systems in Alzheimer's disease. In R. Katzman, R. Terry, & K. Bick (Eds.), *Alzheimer's disease: Senile dementia and related disorders.* New York: Raven Press, 1978.

DeVries, H.A., & Adams, G.M. Electromyographic comparison of single doses of exercise and meprobamate as to effects on muscular relaxation. *American Journal of Physical Medicine,* 1972, *51,* 130-141.

Diesfeldt, H.F.A., & Diesfeldt-Groenendyk, H. Improving cognitive performance in psychogeriatric patients: The influence of physical exercise. *Age and Aging,* 1977, *6,* 58-64.

Dovenmuehle, R.H., & Verwoerdt, A. Physical illness and depression symptomatology, II: Factors of length and severity of illness and frequency of hospitalization. *Journal of Gerontology,* 1963, *18,* 260-266.

Drew, L.R. Alcoholism as a self-limiting disease. *Quarterly Journal of Studies on Alcohol,* 1968, *29* (4), 956-967.

Duckworth, G., & Ross, H. Diagnostic differences in psychogeriatric patients in Toronto, New York, London. *Canadian Medical Association Journal,* 1975, *112,* 847-851.

Durkheim, E. *Suicide.* New York: The Free Press, 1951.

Eisdorfer, C. Paranoia and schizophrenic disorders in later life. In E.W. Busse & D.G. Blazer (Eds.), *Handbook of geriatric psychiatry.* New York: Van Nostrand Reinhold, 1980.

Eisdorfer, C., Nowlin, J., & Wilkie, F. Improvement of learning in the aged by modification of autonomic nervous system activity. *Science,* 1970, *170,* 1327-1329.

Eisdorfer, C., & Stotsky, B.A. Intervention, treatment and rehabilitation of psychiatric disorders. In J.E. Birren & K.W. Schaie (Eds.), *Handbook of the psychology of aging.* New York: Van Nostrand Reinhold, 1977.

Engel, G. *Psychological development in health and disease.* Philadelphia: Saunders, 1962.

Epstein, L.J. Symposium on age differentiation in depressive illness. *Journal of Gerontology,* 1976, *31* (3), 278-282.

Ernst, P., Badask, D., Beran, B., Kosovsky, R., & Kleinhauz, M. Incidence of mental illness in the aged: Unmasking the effects of a diagnosis of chronic brain syndrome. *Journal of the American Geriatric Society,* 1977, *25,* 371-375.

Flavell, J.H. Cognitive changes in adults. In N. Goulet & P. Baltes (Eds.), *Life span developmental psychology research and theory.* New York: Academic Press, 1970.

Folstein, M.F., Folstein, S.E., & McHugh, P.R. "Mini-mental state": A practical method for grading the cognitive state of patients for the clinicians. *Journal of Psychiatric Research,* 1975, *12,* 189-198.

Geriatric medicine: A statement from the Federated Council for Internal Medicine. *Annals of Internal Medicine,* 1981, *95,* 372-376.

Geriscope. *Geriatrics,* 1972, *27,* 120-125.

Glatt, M.M., & Rosin, A.J. Aspects of alcoholism in the elderly. *Lancet,* 1964, *2,* 472-473.

Goldfarb, A.I. Geriatric psychiatry. In A.M. Freeman & H.I. Kaplan (Eds.), *Comprehensive textbook of psychiatry.* Baltimore: Williams & Wilkins, 1967.

Gomberg, E.S. Prevalence of alcoholism among ward patients in a Veterans Administration hospital. *Journal of Studies on Alcohol,* 1975, *36,* 1458-1467.

Gomberg, E.S. Women with alcohol problems. In N.G. Estes & M.E. Heinemann (Eds.), *Alcoholism: Development, consequences and interventions.* St. Louis: C.V. Mosby, 1977.

Gomberg, E.S. Drinking and problem drinking among the elderly. In *Alcohol, drugs and aging: Usage and problems* (Publication No. 1). Ann Arbor: University of Michigan, Institute of Gerontology, 1980.

Gurland, B.J. The comparative frequency of depression in various adult age groups. *Journal of Gerontology,* 1976, *31* (3), 283-292.

Harper, A.E. Recommended dietary allowances for the elderly. *Geriatrics,* May 1978, pp. 73-75; 79-80.

Hausmann, C. Short-term counseling groups for people with elderly parents. *Gerontologist,* 1979, *19,* 102-107.

Hollister, L. An overview of strategies for the development of an effective treatment for senile dementia. In T. Crook & S. Gershon (Eds.), *Strategies for the development of an effective treatment for senile dementia.* New Canaan, Conn.: Mark Powley Associates, 1981.

Jellinger, K. Neuropathological aspects of dementia resulting from abnormal blood and cerebrospinal fluid dynamics. *ACTA Neurology Belgium,* 1976, *76,* 83-102.

Kahn, R.L., Goldfarb, A.I., Pollack, M., & Peck, A. Brief objective measures for the determination of mental status in the aged. *American Journal of Psychiatry,* 1960, *117,* 326-330.

Kahn, R.L., Zarit, S.H., Hilbert, N.M., & Niederehe, G. Memory complaints and impairments in the aged. *Archives of General Psychiatry,* 1975, *32,* 1569-1573.

Katzman, R. The prevalence and malignancy of Alzheimer's disease: A major killer. *Archives of Neurology,* 1976, *33,* 217-218.

Kiloh, L.G. Pseudodementia. *ACTA Psychiatric Scandinavian,* 1961, *37,* 336-351.

Kinsey, A.C., Pomeroy, W.B., & Martin, C.R. *Sexual behavior in the human male.* Philadelphia: W.B. Saunders, 1948.

Klatzo, I., Wisniewski, H., & Streicher, E. Experimental production of neurofibrillary degeneration. *Journal of Neuropathology and Experimental Neurology*, 1965, *24*, 187-199.

Klisz, D. Neuropsychological evaluation in older persons. In M. Storandt, M. Elias, & I. Siegles (Eds.), *The clinical psychology of aging*. New York: Plenum Press, 1978.

Kral, V.A. Benign senescent forgetfulness. In R. Katzman, R. Terry, & K. Bick (Eds.), *Alzheimer's disease: Senile dementia and related disorders*. New York: Raven Press, 1978.

LaBarge, E. Counseling patients with senile dementia of the Alzheimer's type and their families. *The Personnel and Guidance Journal*, November 1981, pp. 139-143.

Libow, L.S. Senile dementia and "pseudonsenility": Clinical investigations by appropriate laboratory tests and a new mental status evaluation technique. In C. Eisdorfer & R. Friedel (Eds.), *Cognitive and emotional disturbances in the elderly: Clinical issues*. Chicago: Year Book Medical Publishers, 1977.

Lieberman, A., Dziatolowsky, M., & Kupersmith, M. Dementia in Parkinson's disease. *Annals of Neurology*, 1979, *6*, 335-359.

Lowenthal, M.F., Berkman, P.L., & associates. *Aging and mental disorders in San Francisco: A social psychiatric study*. San Francisco: Jossey-Bass, 1967.

Mace, N.L., & Rabins, P.V. *The 36-hour day: A family guide to caring for persons with Alzheimer's disease, related dementing illnesses and memory loss in later life*. Baltimore: The Johns Hopkins University Press, 1982.

MacMahon, B., & Pugh, T. Suicide in the widow. *American Journal of Epidemiology*, 1965, *81*, 23-31.

Madorsky, M.L., Ashamalla, M.G., Schussler, I., Lyons, H.R., & Miller, G.H. Post-prostatectomy impotence. *The Journal of Urology*, 1976, *115*, 401-403.

Marden, P.G. *Alcohol abuse and the aged* (Paper No. NCAI026923), Washington, D.C.: National Institute on Alcohol Abuse and Alcoholism, 1976.

Marsden, C.D., & Harrison, M.J. Outcome of investigation in patients with presenile dementia. *British Medical Journal*, 1972, *2*, 249-252.

Masters, W.H., & Johnson, V.E. *Human sexual inadequacy*. London: J.A. Churchill, 1970.

Mendlewicz, J. The age factors in depressive illness: Some genetic considerations. *Journal of Gerontology*, 1976, *31* (3) 300-303.

Meyer, A. The life chart. In Alfred Lief (Ed.), *The common sense psychiatry of Dr. Adolf Meyer*. New York: McGraw-Hill Book Company, 1948.

Miller, N. The measurement of mood in senile brain disease: Examiner ratings and self reports. In J. Cole & J. Barret (Eds.), *Psychopathology in the aged*. New York: Raven Press, 1980.

Morrant, J.C.A. Medicines and mental illnesses in old age. *Canadian Psychiatric Association Journal*, 1975, *20*, 309-312.

National Institute on Aging Task Force. Senility reconsidered: Treatment possibilities for mental impairments in the elderly. *Journal of American Medical Association*, 1980, *244* (3), 259-263.

Neugarten, B.L., & Gutmann, D.L. Age-sex roles and personality in middle age: A thematic apperception study. In B.L. Neugarten (Ed.), *Middle age and aging: A reader in social psychology*. Chicago: University of Chicago Press, 1968.

Newman, G., & Nichols, C.B. Sexual activities and attitudes in older persons. *Journal of American Medical Association*, 1960, *173*, 33-35.

O'Rourke, M. *Elder abuse: The state of the art*. Paper prepared for the National Conference on the Abuse of Older Persons, Boston, March 23-25, 1981; San Francisco, April 1-3, 1981. Boston: Legal Research and Services for the Elderly, 1981.

Pascarelli, E.F. Drug dependence: An age-old problem compounded by old age. *Geriatrics*, 1974, *29*, 109-115.

Pascarelli, E.F., & Fisher, W. Drug dependence in the elderly. *International Journal of Aging and Human Development*, 1974, *5* (4), 347-356.

Pfeiffer, E. A short portable mental status questionnaire for the assessment of organic brain deficit in elderly patients. *Journal of American Geriatric Society*, 1975, *23*, 433-441.

Piaget, J. Intellectual evolution from adolescence to adulthood. *Human Development*, 1972, *15*, 1-12.

Post, F. The significance of affective symptoms in old age. *Maudsley Monographs No. 10*. London: Oxford University Press, 1962.

Raskind, M., & Eisdorfer, C. Psychopharmacology of the aged. In L.L. Simpson (Ed.), *Drug treatment of mental disorders*. New York: Raven Press, 1976.

Raskind, M., & Storrie, M.C. The organic mental disorders. In E. Busse & D. Blazer (Eds.), *Handbook of geriatric psychiatry*. New York: Van Nostrand Reinhold, 1980.

Rathbone-McCuan, E., Lohn, H., Levenson, J., & Hsu, J. *Community survey of aged alcoholics and problem drinkers* (National Technical Information Service, Pub. No. 1R18-AA, 01734-01). Baltimore: Levindale Geriatric Research Center, National Institute on Alcohol Abuse and Alcoholism, 1976.

Rathbone-McCuan, E., & Triegaardt, J. *The older alcoholic and the family*. Paper presented at the National Council on Alcoholism, St. Louis, 1978.

Reading, A. The role of the general hospital in a community alcoholism program. *Proceedings of the 3rd Annual Alcoholism Conference*, National Institute on Alcohol Abuse and Alcoholism, 1974, 254-266.

Reiff, T.R. The essentials of a geriatric evaluation. *Geriatrics*, May 1980, pp. 59-62; 67-68.

Reisberg, B., & Ferris, S.H. Diagnosis and assessment of the older patient. *Hospital and Community Psychiatry*, 1982, *33* (2), 104-110.

Resnick, H.L., & Cantor, J.M. Suicide and aging. *Journal of the American Geriatric Society*, 1970, *18*, 152-158.

Rich, J.A., & Eyde, D.R. *Assessment of insight in the cognitively impaired elderly*. Paper presented at the 33rd Annual Scientific Meeting of the Gerontological Society of America. Toronto, Canada, November 21-25, 1980. *Gerontologist II*, 1980, *20* (5), 186.

Rich, J.A., & Eyde, D.R. A matrix approach to cognition and aging. *Perspectives in adult learning and development*. May 1981.

Rowe, J.W. Research in geriatrics and gerontology. In A. Somers & D. Fabian (Eds.), *The geriatric imperative: An introduction to gerontology and clinical geriatrics*. New York: Appleton-Century-Crofts, 1981.

Schaie, K.W. Psychological changes from midlife to early old age: Implications for the maintenance of mental health. *American Journal of Orthopsychiatry*, 1981, *51*, 199-218.

Schmidt, W., & de Lint, J. Mortality experiences of male and female alcoholic patients. *Quarterly Journal of Studies on Alcohol*, 1969, *30*, 112-118.

Schneck, M.K., Reisberg, B., & Ferris, S.H. An overview of current concepts of Alzheimer's disease. *American Journal of Psychiatry*, 1982, *139* (2), 165-173.

Schuckit, M.A. Geriatric alcoholism and drug abuse. *Gerontologist*, 1977, *17*, 168-174.

Schuckit, M.A., & Pastor, P.A. The elderly as a unique population: Alcoholism. *Alcoholism, Clinical and Experimental Research*, 1978, *2*, 31-38.

Seligman, M.E. *Helplessness: On depression, development and death.* San Francisco: W.H. Freeman, 1975.

Shock, N.W. Biological theories of aging. In J.E. Birren & K.W. Schaie (Eds.), *Handbook of the psychology of aging.* New York: Van Nostrand Reinhold Co., 1977.

Sigurdsson, B. Rida, a chronic encephalitis of sheep with general remarks on infections which develop slowly and some of their special characteristics. *British Veterinarian Journal,* 1954, *110,* 341–343.

Snyder, V. Aging, alcoholism, and reactions to loss. *Social Work,* 1977, *22,* 232–233.

Sparacino, J. An attributional approach to psychotherapy with the aged. *Journal of American Geriatrics Society,* 1978, *26,* 9–13.

Sternberg, D.E., & Jarvik, M.E. Memory functions in depression. *Archives of General Psychiatry,* 1976, *33,* 219–224.

Straus, M.A., Gelles, R., & Steinmetz, S. *Behind closed doors.* Garden City, New York: Anchor/Doubleday, 1980.

Subby, P. *A community based program for the chemically dependent elderly.* Paper presented at North American Congress on Alcohol and Drug Problems, San Francisco, December 1975.

Sweet, R.D., McDowell, F.H., Feigenson, J.S., et al. Mental symptoms in Parkinson's disease during chronic treatment with levodopa. *Neurology,* 1976, *26,* 305–310.

Task Force on Prescription Drugs. *The drug users.* Washington, D.C.: U.S. Government Printing Office, 1968.

Tkach, J.R., & Hokama, Y. Autoimmunity in chronic brain syndrome: A preliminary report. *Archives of General Psychology,* 1970, *23,* 61–64.

Todhunter, E.N., & Darby, W.J. Guidelines for maintaining adequate nutrition in old age. *Geriatrics,* June 1978, pp. 49–51; 54–56.

Tomlinson, B.E., Blessed, J., & Roth, M. Observations on the brains of demented old people. *Journal of the Neurological Sciences,* 1970, *11,* 205–242.

Verwoerdt, A. Individual psychotherapy in senile dementia. In N. Miller & G. Cohen (Eds.), *Clinical aspects of Alzheimer's disease and senile dementia (Aging,* Vol. 15). New York: Raven Press, 1981.

Wang, J.A., & Whanger, A. Brain impairments and longevity. In E. Palmore & F. Jeffers (Eds.), *Prediction of life span.* Lexington, Mass.: D.C. Heath, 1971.

Weiler, P., & Rathbone-McCuan, E. *Adult day care: Community work with the elderly.* New York: Springer Publishing, 1978.

Wells, C.E. Dementia: Definition and description. In C.E. Wells (Ed.), *Dementia* (2nd ed.). Philadelphia: F.A. Davis, 1977.

Wells, C.E. Chronic brain disease: An overview. *American Journal of Psychiatry,* 1978, *135,* 1–12.

Wells, C.E. Management of dementia. In R. Katzman (Ed.), *Congenital and acquired cognitive disorders.* New York: Raven Press, 1979.

Wells, C.E. Chronic brain disease: An update on alcoholism, Parkinson's disease and dementia. *Hospital and Community Psychiatry,* 1982, *33* (2), 111–126.

Winokur, G. Genetic and clinical factors associated with course in depression. *Pharmakopsychiatry, Neuropsychopharmakol,* 1974, *7,* 122–126.

Winokur, G., Morrison, J., Clancy, J., & Crowe, R. The Iowa 500: Familiar and clinical families favor two kinds of depressive illness. *Comprehensive Psychiatry,* 1973, *14,* 99–107.

Zimberg, S. The elderly alcoholic. *Gerontologist,* 1974, *14,* 221–224.

Chapter 6

Community-Based Services: Issues, Trends, and Future Challenges

ISSUES IN DELIVERY OF SERVICES

The current and anticipated impact of demographic changes on community, state, and federal resources is increasingly becoming a point of public policy debate. In 1981, 5 percent of the gross national product and 24 percent of federal expenditures were related to the care needs of the elderly. Consumption of social and health care resources are expected to increase to 10 percent and 40 percent respectively as the postwar "baby boom" becomes the "senior boom" (Califano, 1981).

State and federal agencies have responded to the "aging problem" by constructing an array of programs and policies aptly termed by Estes (1979) "the aging enterprise." This "aging enterprise" initially grew from policy makers' concern for appropriate health care for dependent elderly and is reflected in the enactment of Medicare (Title XVIII) and Medicaid (Title XIX). The decade of the 1970s witnessed increased concern for social programs as well as medical needs of the aged. The passage of Title XX of the Social Security Act, Title III of the Older Americans Act, and related legislation was aimed at reducing inappropriate placement of individuals in institutions by providing community-based resources and home-centered alternatives. (Appendix 6-A presents an interview with Evelyn Runyon, ombudsman and director of supportive services with the Eastern Nebraska Office on Aging, regarding issues, trends, and future challenges of these resources and alternatives.)

While policy makers rhetorically shifted community-based health and social programs, the service models were still heavily skewed toward acute medically oriented health care. For example, Estes (1979) reports that in 1978, the Department of Health, Education, and Welfare expended $94 billion for programs to serve the aged, including Medicare and Medicaid, but less than 5 percent of those expenditures was allocated for community-based health and social services. Butler (1979) notes that while 1.7 to 2.7 million older individuals need home health care and day care, only 300,000 to 500,000 receive it through formal mechanisms. The legislative approach to meeting the health and social care needs of the elderly has, in fact, created a set of fragmented, discontinuous services that bewilder. Califano (1981) notes that three areas of concern continue to cycle throughout most discussion about the aging problem: (1) the adequacy of definitions of old age and retirement, (2) income security, and (3) the provision of social and health care services. All three policy questions have significant import for the aged and their families; however, the most pressing concerns are the delivery, location, and cost of social health care services.

The "continuum of care" movement summarizes these concerns. The implication of the continuum of care approach is that a decision as to relative dependency and relative need should be made, and then a service package utilizing a variety of care options should be designed to match the need. At one end of the continuum may be an older person who is somewhat compromised, perhaps because a driver's license has been revoked, but other than transportation, does not require extensive assistance. Further along the continuum may be functionally impaired elderly who need support and assistance with daily living activities in order to stay in their own home. At the extreme of the continuum may be the fully dependent impaired older person who requires so many specialized services to survive that it is most cost-effective to place the person in an environment where the services are routinely available such as in a general-care, intermediate-care, or long-term facility (McCuan, Lohn, Levenson & Hsu, 1975). Certainly exercising this latter option has led to the expansion of the nursing home industry and inappropriate placement of older persons out of the community. Nursing home costs, for example, accounted for 40 cents of every Medicare dollar spent in 1981.

It is relatively easy to describe the continuum, its content, and its environmental context as Califano (1981) observes:

> Such a system would include: (1) adequate and supervised residential facilities for those who lack families but want to live in their community; (2) special services for those who live at home but need help from the outside, for example, help with transportation, shopping and help with meals and personal care; (3) a range of alternatives between the hospital and the nursing home including a system of home health care; and (4) innovative and compassionate ways of caring for the terminally ill outside the traditional hospital or nursing home. (p. 289)

Appropriate community-based support services along the continuum then should possess the following characteristics: they should be multifaceted with biological, psychological, and social components; they should provide a response to specific needs of the elderly, available as close to natural environments as possible; and they should be coordinated, available, and acceptable. Such services should encompass a spectrum of need from promoting and maintaining health to preventing and care for disease and disability (Myers & Drayer, 1979).

Dr. Klerman (1980, p. 81) testified that among the prominent barriers to improving delivery of mental health care services for the elderly are the following: benefit levels for mental health reimbursement in public and private insurance plans that promote inappropriate placement and discourage other modes of care; inadequate training and availability of personnel leading to inadequate diagnosis and care programs; negative attitude toward treatability of mental health problems in the aged; inadequate coordination of services once needs are identified; lack or availability of community care; and negative attitudes of the elderly toward mental health needs, which prevents many from seeking timely care.

The structure of Medicare reimbursements is a continual barrier to the development and utilization of community-based services. Medicare limits reimbursements of inpatient psychiatric treatment to 190 days during a person's lifetime and puts a ceiling of $250 per year in most states on the use of outpatient psychiatric services. This type of restrictive financing encourages the use of state hospitals and nursing homes as service locations. In essence, a lack of understanding of the nature and treatment of later-life mental disorders on the part of professionals, the elderly themselves, and their families undermines the realization of a true continuum of care in most communities. Maddox (1980) argues that the establishment of a continuum of community-based service is really not the issue. However, the effectiveness and efficiency of these services "continues to be asserted rather than demonstrated" (p. 501). The problem is that available service packages are typically not coordinated and not routinely accessed or accessible by a majority of older individuals or their families.

TRENDS IN DELIVERY OF COMMUNITY SERVICES FOR THE AGED

Despite the restrictiveness of reimbursable care options, a number of community alternatives are evolving. Over the past two decades, the concept of the *social network* has evolved from a metaphor into a process of service delivery termed *networking* (Cohen & Sokolovsky, 1979). Networking has become an important consideration in clinical assessment as well as for planning decisions related to service delivery. A network is a specific set of linkage among a set of people, such that the characteristics of the linkage as a whole may be used to understand and possibly to predict the social behavior of the whole (Mitchell, 1969). Lopata (1975) states that the connections between people characterized by the giving and receiving of objects, services, and social and emotional support necessary to maintaining a style of life may be understood as a "support system."

Support systems and socioemotional linkages are apparently important in maintaining mental and physical health, particularly in the elderly (Clark & Anderson, 1967; Gruenberg, 1954; Lowenthal, 1964; Williams & Jaco, 1958). Physical wellness and susceptibility to disease likewise have been correlated with social support systems (Berkman, 1978; Cassel, 1973; Rabkin & Struening, 1976). Authors such as Cohen and Sokolovsky (1979) are studying the context as parameters of supportive transactions, the content of these relationships, and the linkages between networks. Their research illuminates data that should be an important consideration for planners of formal services.

Cohen and Sokolovsky (1979) suggest that service providers first determine what primary network strengths and weaknesses exist and what "second-order" linkages are available. Second-order relationships consist of individuals indirectly linked with the individual network such as a "friend-of-a-friend." Secondly, agency personnel should determine whether the provision of formal services would, in fact, interfere with the less formal network of support. Lastly, agencies must ascertain if components or formal and informal support are contradictory and in conflict. For example, if one agency may be providing meals at home to preserve independence and the other may be arranging for nursing home placement, socioemotional assistance, e.g., network therapy (Speck & Attneave, 1973) and physical assistance should be sought first from the individual, "natural" support group. Formal services may actually interfere with extant services provided by the informal network system.

The consequences of disrupting social networks, particularly changing locality, are pervasive (Fried, 1963). Aldrich and Mendhoff (1963) report high rates of depression and mortality following relocation of the elderly and subsequent loss of social buffer zones that might have lessened the trauma. Hochschild (1973) demonstrates a similar finding in studies of housing projects and the linkages of mutual assistance. Several authors suggest the importance of elderly self-help groups and familiar environments in maintenance of psychological well-being (Hess, 1976; Petty, Moeller, & Campbell, 1976).

Self-help groups for families of the elderly oriented toward specific needs or experiences are also evident in the natural community (Collins & Pancoast, 1976). The family support group for victims of Alzheimer's and related disorders found throughout the country is one such example. These groups provide information and advocacy services, share strategies for survival, and generally provide the sense that someone else has gone through it too. The popularity of these groups suggests that professionals may not be responding adequately to the distress that impairments cause in first- and second-order network relationships.

Preservation of meaningful social connection within an individual's network is necessary to one's well-being. Even nursing homes are beginning to appreciate and support the importance of maintaining or initiating an affective bridge to the community. In-home care services are also rapidly expanding along with specialized geriatric daycare centers. However, many elderly, because of the stigma of charity, do not access these services. The psychology of "entitlements" has not saturated the thinking of the elderly in the same way as it has permeated current attitudes of others (Trunzo, 1982). Home-care services that may be obtained include nursing care, occupational and physical therapy, and home-making services, including shopping, meal preparation, and help with daily hygiene and home repairs. Outreach programs involving mental health teams for the seriously cognitively impaired elderly are also available in certain areas (Reifler, Kethley, O'Neill, Hanley, Lewis, & Stenchever, 1982). However, barriers continue to prevent full utilization of community and in-home services, especially mental health services (Hagebak & Hagebak, 1980).

FUTURE CHALLENGES: TEACHING FAMILIES DECISION MAKING

Long-term care, unfortunately, has become synonymous with nursing homes or institutional placement whereas the true goal of long-term care is for people to receive the right services at the right time in the most appropriate place, based on their needs (English, 1981). Acute care emphasizes cure or improvement in episodic illness. Long-term care should include therapeutic rehabilitation to improve functioning and efforts to maintain current levels of functioning as well as protective care where appropriate. Long-term care should have a sense of continuity or continuous delivery of appropriate services offered on a continuum that integrates, not polarizes, community-based and institutional services. Families particularly have suffered from the semantic errors of "long-term care" as they anguish over institutional placement of an older member in order to gain access to a certain cluster of health and social services.

Dworkin (1972) notes that "to be able to choose is a good that is independent from the wisdom of what is chosen" (p. 75). Families in the past often did not have a workable decision-making model to help them choose. Forced choices become, in fact, no choices.

The philosophical extension of community-based mental health services fortunately is changing this state of affairs. Community mental health treatment programs, according to Northman (1978), acknowledge social treatment goals that were designed to aid the individual achieve social adjustment in ordinary life situations. Ordinary life includes the individual's place within a family system. Secondly, community health treatment recognizes "problems in living" that were deficient in environmental supports, not deficits in personality structure. Consequently, the environmental context of family became increasingly significant as a "natural support system." It was discovered that the family was in the best position to assure that continuous care services were delivered to the individual member in need. Moreover, the family could function as a "systematic integrator," coordinating services and assistance between subsystems. Increased decision-making responsibility was located within the family system as a result of these rediscoveries. The professional began to function as a broker, and the family had to assume the burden of guilt and remorse as out-of-home placement/long-term care plans were initiated.

Currently, community-based brokers are more active in helping families with decision-making chores. The connection between assessment and placement is being clarified along three important dimensions: (1) type of service needed, (2) amount (intensity) of service, and (3) location of services and necessary living situations (English, 1981). The research of Pfeiffer, Johnson, and Chiofolo (1981) demonstrates that the functional status of impaired elderly, assessment of the appropriateness of services provided, and determination of unmet services are needed before recommendations are made either for changes in services provided within the site or for transfer to a more appropriate service setting.

Families should be helped to determine accurately what the care and assistance needs of older members are, what services and support including family can be utilized, what the needs of other family members are, and how these needs can be prioritized. Fortunately, more and more families are being encouraged to do more proactive anticipatory planning that involves taking into account the older person's preferences, clearing up unfinished business, and reviewing the system of old promises for support and assistance that may be applicable to the current situation.

The family is the client in modern community-based services; Szasz's (1956) "model of mutual participation" is being frequently utilized to provide more authority and control to the family and older member since they are generally better able to determine what is needed more accurately than the professional. On an ethical level, two major issues arise from increased family participation in decision making: (1) autonomy versus paternalism, and (2) rights of individual privacy (Sorensen, 1981). Paternalism is "the interference with a person's liberty of action justified by reasons referring exclusively to the welfare, good, happiness, interests or values of the person" (Dworkin, 1972, p. 65) whose choices are usurped. Autonomy in this context suggests that the person has the right to sufficient information to make informed choices. The second issue of privacy involves the individual's right to control intimate personal data and determine who should have access to that information. Confidentiality and the right to bodily integrity are part of the overall right-to-privacy issue. It has been shown that in cases where these rights are continuously violated, the individual may seek more primitive levels of control by withdrawing into oneself and consequently may redefine the self that is being violated. While family participation is encouraged, these ethical issues must also be considered.

The older person should participate to the maximum extent practical in every decision that involves his or her physical and socioemotional well-being. Otherwise the very process of family decision making becomes another arena of loss for the older person.

As one last note, locating resources in the community may not be easy; patience and persistence are the watchwords. Many telephone calls and visits to service agencies such as the health and welfare departments, United Way, Red Cross, or information and referral services at local, county, or state levels of government may be necessary. The Public Affairs Committee, Inc. (Irwin, 1978) published the following checklist, which might aid in organization of service search missions.

Community Services Checklist

Are the following resources for the elderly available in your community?
Transportation and/or escort services
A senior center offering social activities and recreation
Group meals program in a social setting
A day center for the elderly
Library, museum, and performing arts programs
Adult education opportunities
Job opportunities and/or senior citizens employment service
Volunteer opportunities and/or senior talent pool
Legal and general counseling
A local council on aging
A "senior power" activist organization
An information and referral center for the aging
In-home services such as:

- Visiting nurse service
- Homemaker-home health aides
- Telephone reassurance
- Friendly visiting
- Meals on Wheels

REFERENCES

Aldrich, C., & Mendhoff, E. Relocation of the aged and disabled: A mortality study. *Journal of the American Geriatrics Society*, 1963, *11* (3), 401–408.

Berkman, L. Social isolation shortens lives. *Medical World News*, January 8, 1978, p. 13.

Butler, P. Financing non-institutional long term care services for the elderly and chronically ill: Alternatives to nursing homes. *Clearing-house Review*, September 1979.

Califano, J.A. The aging of America and the four generation society. In R.B. Hudson (Ed.), *The aging in politics: Process and policy*. Springfield, Ill.: Charles C. Thomas, 1981.

Cassel, J. The relation of the urban environment to health: Implications for prevention. *Mount Sinai Journal of Medicine*, 1973, *40*, 539–550.

Clark, M., & Anderson, B.G. *Culture and aging: An anthropological study of older Americans*. Springfield, Ill.: Charles C. Thomas, 1967.

Cohen, C.I., & Sokolovsky, J. Clinical use of network analysis for psychiatric and aged populations. *Community Mental Health Journal*, 1979, *15* (3), 203–213.

Collins, A., & Pancoast, D.L. *Natural helping networks*. Washington, D.C.: National Association of Social Workers, 1976,

Dworkin, G. Paternalism. *Monist*, 1972, *56*, 64–84.

English, N. Long-term care in the community. In G. Sorenson (Ed.), *Older persons and service providers: An instructor's training guide*. New York: Human Sciences Press, 1981.

Estes, C.L. *The aging enterprise*. San Francisco: Jossey-Bass, 1979.

Fried, M. Grieving for a lost home. In L. Duhl (Ed.), *The urban condition*. New York: Basic Books, 1963.

Gruenberg, E. Community conditions and psychosis of the elderly. *American Journal of Psychiatry*, 1954, *110*, 888–896.

Hagebak, J.E., & Hagebak, B.R. Serving the mental health needs of the elderly: The case for removing barriers and improving service integration. *Community Mental Health Journal*, 1980, *16* (4), 263–275.

Hatch, O.G. Home health care: Necessary option for older Americans. *Hospital Progress*, April 1981, pp. 6–10.

Hess, B.B. Self-help among the aged. *Social Policy*, November/ December 1976, pp. 55–62.

Hochschild, A. *The unexpected community*. Englewood Cliffs, N.J.: Prentice-Hall, 1973.

Irwin, T. *After 65: Resources for self-reliance* (Public Affairs Pamphlet No. 501 Special Ed.). Rockville, Md.: U.S. Department of Health, Education, and Welfare, National Institute of Mental Health, Alcohol, Drug Abuse and Mental Health Administration, 1978.

Klerman, G.L. Prepared statement. *In Aging and mental health: Overcoming barriers to service* (Commerce Publication No. 67–899–0). Hearing before the Special Committee on Aging, U.S. Senate, Ninety-Sixth Congress, Second Session, Part 2, Washington D.C.: U.S. Government Printing Office, May 22, 1980.

Lopata, H. Support systems of elderly: Chicago of the 1970's. *Gerontologist*, 1975, *15*, 35–41.

Lowenthal, M.F. Social isolation and mental illness in old age. *American Sociological Review*, 1964, *29*, 54–70.

Maddox, G.L. The continuum of care: Movement toward the community. In E.W. Busse and D.G. Blazer (Eds.), *Handbook of geriatric psychiatry*. New York: Van Nostrand Reinhold, 1980.

Manney, J. *Aging in American Society*. Ann Arbor, Mich.: Institute of Gerontology, 1975.

McCuan, E., Lohn, H., Levenson, J., & Hsu, J. *Cost-effectiveness evaluation of the Levindale adult day treatment centers.* Baltimore: Levindale Geriatric Research Center, 1975.

Mitchell, J.C. Concept and use of social networks. In J.C. Mitchell (Ed.), *Social networks in urban situations.* Manchester, England: Manchester University Press, 1969.

Myers, J.M., & Drayer, C.S. Support systems and mental illness in the elderly. *Community Mental Health Journal,* 1979, *15* (4), 277-286.

Northman, J.E. Human service program design and the family. *Family and Community Health,* 1978, *1* (2), 17-26.

Petty, B.J., Moeller, T.P., & Campbell, R.Z. Support groups for elderly persons in the community. *Gerontologist,* 1976, *15*, 522-527.

Pfeiffer, E., Johnson, T.M., & Chiofolo, R.C. Functional assessment of elderly subjects in four service settings. *Journal of the American Geriatrics Society,* 1981, *29* (10), 433-437.

Pfeiffer, J.W. Conditions which hinder effective communication. In G. Sorensen (Ed.), *Older persons and service providers: An instructor's training guide.* New York: Human Sciences Press, 1981.

Rabkin, J.G., & Struening, E.L. Life events, stress and illness. *Science,* 1976, *194*, 1013-1020.

Reifler, B.V., Kethley, A., O'Neill, P., Hanley, R., Lewis, S., & Stenchever, D. Five-year experience of a community outreach program for the elderly. *American Journal of Psychiatry,* 1982, *139* (2), 220-223.

Riessman, F. *The role of self-help groups in the mental health field.* Paper presented at the annual meeting of the American Psychiatric Association, Atlanta, May 1978.

Sorensen, G. The ethics of helping. In G. Sorensen (Ed.), *Older persons and service providers: An instructor's training guide.* New York: Human Sciences Press, 1981.

Speck, R.V., & Attneave, C.L. *Family Networks.* New York: Pantheon, 1973.

Szasz, T., & Hollendar, M. The basic models of the doctor-patient relationship. *Archives in Internal Medicine,* 1956, *97*, 585-592.

Trunzo, C.E. Solving the age-old problem. *Money,* January 1982, pp. 70-72; 74; 76; 78.

Williams, W.S., & Jaco, E.G. An evaluation of functional psychoses in old age. *American Journal of Psychiatry,* 1958, *114*, 910-916.

Appendix 6-A

An Interview with Evelyn Runyon

Dr. Rich: It has been argued that community-based alternatives to nursing homes are available but they are fragmented, uncoordinated, and often inaccessible to a majority of the elderly who need them. From your perspective as ombudsman and director of supportive services with the Eastern Nebraska Office on Aging, would you first describe the types of information, referral, and support services typically available from an area Office on Aging and then comment on Manney's [1975] specific concerns?

Evelyn Runyon: There should be no limit to the number of sources of services and referrals. It is up to the ombudsman to find a source that will fulfill the necessary referral. It may not be a formal one and it may not be a generally known one. But somewhere, somehow, if there were a capability of fulfilling the need at all, the resources of the ombudsman should create some way to find whatever is needed to fulfill that need. Sometimes it takes a long time. I remember one case where I worked for almost six months to get the proper referral, but in the meantime I also do remember that some other needs became evident. I was able to take care of some of the contributing factors in the overall need. It takes a lot of resourcefulness sometimes and a lot of study.

Rich: What are the typical support services?

Runyon: The *basic* support services are such things as nutrition (either a meal site or home delivery of meals), homemakers, handymen, transportation, some support in untangling financial and legal affairs—these are *basic*. They usually denote an immediate need and also a need that is not the basic or the immediate need of that individual. They are basic services offered in response to general symptoms.

For example, when older persons call to ask for the closest nutrition site and how to get there and how much does it cost, that only tells me that there are

176

some needs. In other words, are they alone in the home? Do they or don't they like to cook or can't they cook or are they having trouble getting groceries? Have they recently lost someone with whom they ate? Is it that they just don't want to stay at home at mealtime? The request for basic service opens up the need for more complete review.

The ombudsman and information and referral people have a responsibility to figure out what goes beyond the basic. The basic services are rare enough.

Rich: Manney [1975] cited the following reasons: (1) particular services are unavailable, (2) services are fragmented, (3) the elderly lack information about availability of the services, (4) services are inaccessible because of red tape and roadblocks within the service delivery system, and (5) services are impersonalized.

Do you find that particular services are unavailable?

Runyon: That should be a very rare occasion, because if the agency providing services cannot find that service someplace, then that agency needs to reevaluate its purpose. For instance, let's say that there is no meal site. The first thing that I would want to do would be to call the church and find out if it has meals of any kind at any time. If not, then the next thing I would want to do would be to find out if there are some groups within the neighborhood, maybe a bridge club. Very often neighbors can be found who will prepare a meal. At other times, another service such as a homemaker could go in and cook a meal for the person. If a basic service is unavailable, there should be a commitment, energy, and resourcefulness in finding a viable substitute.

Rich: Do you find that the services are fragmented?

Runyon: Services are fragmented, but this should not be so. If the caregiver understands case management, then there must be a way of integrating the services so as to make them not seem fragmented. But it is true that this depends on the ingenuity of the caregiver to keep the fragmentation from being apparent.

Rich: Do the elderly lack information about the availability of services?

Runyon: That is absolutely true, but there should be some resource where older people can obtain the information. Of course, that is really the responsibility of the sponsoring agency through an information and referral service. If we could make sure that older people could know that there is an information and referral service, then we would overcome that deficiency.

Usually the elderly look for information about available services through their churches and community groups. It behooves the agency to have a good active working relationship with the ministerial groups in any community and to have a clear and solid public image among other community groups.

The media is good for general information, but person-to-person information really needs to come through an individual such as a minister or community leader.

Rich: Are services inaccessible because of red tape and roadblocks within the service delivery system?

Runyon: Yes, however, we are beginning to overcome these. All the work of agencies is beginning to create an understanding that there do not need to be roadblocks. The roadblocks are being wiped out to some extent and will be more so.

One of the bigger roadblocks is that workers have not realized that they can ask for cooperation. One of the main roadblocks is territoriality; that is being gradually done away with in a spirit of cooperation.

Rich: Are services impersonalized?

Runyon: Unfortunately, this seems so and I am sorry to have to say that. Human services demand the human touch, and services for older people should not be impersonal. The difficulty with impersonal services is in choosing workers. A skillful worker will never seem impersonal. If agencies would make sure that skills had been learned or had been acquired by the worker in human services, we could enhance services.

Rich: Senator Hatch [1981] recently said that "about 25 percent of the Americans now in nursing homes do not need to be there, but they are forced to enter prematurely because of the way current Medicare/Medicaid laws are written" [p. 6]. Is this an accurate estimate?

Runyon: This is a conservative figure. A great number of people in nursing homes do not have to be there. If it were possible to provide support for home care, we would have fewer people in nursing homes.

Rich: What do you see as the real barriers to maintaining community-based continuity of care?

Runyon: The real barrier is lack of financial support. Medicaid and Medicare support for health service could often be much better spent in home care. We have to realize, too, that Medicare does not provide financial help in nursing homes unless the person needs skilled care and then for only a certain number of days. It falls to either the family or to an intermediate-care facility to care for this person, when in reality it's intermediary care. Then certainly, in many instances, the person could be at home, if there were care at home.

Rich: How can families of the elderly and the elderly themselves overcome the barriers to maintaining community-based care?

Runyon: They can through the agencies that are providing the care, through the information and referral system. Definitely they should be aggressive; certainly in any community there are persons who would know where these services are available. We can't help but hope that community-based options will be positive. It can't come about, however, under the existing regulations. It is going to take financial support for the family who is taking care of the older person at home. In many ways, this is to the advantage of both the older person and the younger family, and it would relieve the burden of financial stress and would keep the person out of a nursing home.

Rich: How will the renewed emphasis on home health legislation affect care options; will the family's role change significantly?

Runyon: The family's role would be so positive that we should pay a great deal more attention to this. Home health care not only provides for the older person in a much more humanistic way, but if there is a younger generation in the family, then the young members should understand what it means to care for an older person. That would be positive; certainly there is a certain deep satisfaction for anyone taking care of a person in need. It would be a positive thing for the daughters and sons and granddaughters and grandsons of the older person to assume whatever responsibility were necessary, with financial support. Home health care would maintain   valuable human relationships.

Rich: According to Riessman [1978], there is a renewal of interest in naturalistic community-based services including indigenous support networks and self-help groups. The continuum of care movement typically has focused on identifying viable alternatives to institutional care; in the process the use of social networks and in-home help has been rediscovered. How is that rediscovery going to affect the older person and their family?

Runyon: The great value of social networks is in maintaining and intensifying the older person's association with the familiar. Finding social networks within the person's own community should include looking in the area where that person is more familiar. In that area there must be some way, somehow, to find a group of individuals who either would know the older person or could help us find some way to get this person involved in something. Sometimes, it is no more than a nutrition site or in some instances maybe a game of bingo. It is important not to transport people from their communities but to be resourceful and imaginative about finding ways to intensify familiar and new associations with others.

Rich: The concepts of special ombudsman, information brokers, channeling professional problem solvers and networking with other care professionals are gaining popularity. What do these concepts mean?

Runyon: They are formal linkages that are a means of making the informal ones possible. These concepts support a need for a full gamut of services and a knowledge of how to and where to plug people in for help.

Rich: What unique services and needs do they meet?

Runyon: They bring linkages to the person in need and provide a monitoring and assessing function. It is important to keep as few services in place as necessary to meet the needs. It is equally important for these brokers, problem solvers, and networkers to fortify the individuals' ability to meet their own needs. In addition it is necessary for care providers to anticipate a time in the future when older persons cannot meet their own need and may have additional needs.

Rich: How do they fit into a continuum of service approaches?

Runyon: They provide the transitions to support services and help older persons develop their potential to meet their own needs.

Rich: Is territoriality or the battle over parts of the problem going to be an issue in community-based versus nursing home services?

Runyon: Definitely territoriality is going to be an issue if there is any financial support for home services. Nursing homes will probably consider and point out the possible inadequacy of home service. If we have home services, then there will be so many things available to the family such as physical therapy, X-ray, and community nursing care, everything that is being supplied in a nursing home setting and even psychological and special therapies. Much of the therapy for people in nursing homes can be done at home. Nursing homes will also argue the issue of 24-hour care. There are bound to be roadblocks that will be thrown up by the nursing home industry for self-preservation.

Rich: Do you anticipate territoriality in current or future home health providers?

Runyon: Yes, that is going to depend on the agency such as a hospital providing home health care. Some hospitals are still limiting the home care to their own staff members, but some others do not have this limitation.

Rich: What additional trends do you perceive in the delivery of community home-based services, including mental health services?

Runyon: The team effort is bound to grow because it is coordinated with the knowledge of available services and their effectiveness. The team effort leads to a plan that integrates all needed services and makes a holistic approach possible.

A team also obscures any emphasis on mental health services that may have a negative connotation for older people. Older persons feel that they would be stigmatized if anybody knew that they were getting mental help of any kind. Within the team, however, mental health remains a significant factor in provision of all services. The label of mental health services is necessary for professionals but it is not palatable for older persons looking at services. The ingenuity and skill of caregivers will be vital in terms of knowledge of the individual, knowledge of the environment, and knowledge of the life-span attachments of the older individual.

Rich: How can family members and elderly go about locating community resources?

Runyon: There is an important need for increased public awareness. Agencies providing services must make themselves known through various means— the media and natural community support groups such as churches, social groups, and service clubs. Services are not available unless families know where they can be found. It is the responsibility of the service providers to increase public awareness. If people know that they can at least try to locate services by calling city officials, law enforcement, police agencies, or existing community resources, they are more likely to find the existing resources. If the network is cooperating, the network makes referrals.

I have been insisting on a speakers' bureau from the networks. The networks should have a speakers' bureau that would actively seek opportunities to explain where the services are and what the services are. Hospitals are a good source of information and referral. At the minimum, the local Area Agency on Aging should be available from the phone book for those seeking services.

Rich: Pfeiffer [1981] identified a number of roadblocks to communication that seem to be operating in the communications and miscommunications between families and professionals including preoccupation, emotional interference, hostility, hidden agendas, lack of verbal skills, and defensiveness. How can families and older persons talk to professionals and get meaningful answers?

Runyon: First of all, the family needs to understand that the professionals are also human, that they are not on a pedestal. There is an awe of professionals that needs to be broken down in some way. In other words, the families should not be afraid of the professional or should not be timid in asking questions or discussing the situation with the professional.

They also need to be sure the person from whom they are seeking answers is knowledgeable and empathetic and has an active desire to help. It is the professional's responsibility to stimulate an active interest among families great enough to maintain an active interaction and persistence in the person asking the question.

In other words, it is necessary for the professionals to have an active desire to help. This desire is made up of a set of skills including listening, counseling, curiosity, and the ability of the professional to eliminate apathy and ambiguity in questions of family members. There needs to be a resourcefulness on the part of the person giving the information. No two individuals are alike enough to give up the need for resourcefulness in providing useful information. The professional must discern the listener's background well enough to know what level of language is understood.

Rich: It has been said that the loss of privacy and loss of freedom are major negative aspects of long-term care options regardless of actual placement [Sorensen, 1981]. What are your feelings regarding the issue of autonomy versus paternalism in family decision making and the individual's right to control personal information and determine who has access to that information?

Runyon: Privacy is of great importance in preserving and strengthening the dignity and sense of self-worth of the older person. If it becomes necessary to relay the information that one has secured, then I would certainly advise discussing this with the older person. An older person must have the maturity to understand the need for sharing information in problem solving. I would ask the older person if he or she minds if we were to talk with another professional, and I would emphasize that the purpose is to help this older person.

All personal relationships relating to any aspect of help should by all means carry the absolute assurance of confidentiality. The older person has always expected this of a physician. It is part of their pattern of thinking that they need that assurance. Certainly privacy has much to do with self-esteem because then you are recognizing the individual as a unique person, that this person is important to you.

Nothing can destroy dignity more effectively than out-and-out paternalism. You are telling the older person that he or she is not capable, and that makes it almost impossible to help the older person in using potential.

Autonomy is vital. Very often autonomy can be given to an older person in the decision-making process with the full knowledge that several recommended actions and procedures would be most helpful and needed. The person planning with the older person should have the skills to build that in so that the older person feels that the decision was his or hers. This also is very important in maintaining dignity and self-esteem and promotes cooperation.

Chapter 7

Promises and Pitfalls of the Family Management Model

The family management model represents a new approach to the complex symptomatology, pathology, and treatments of psychological distress of aging. This model holds the promise of reconnecting and strengthening the quality of relationships between families and their older members. Families can more confidently approach the problems of their older members with added information skills and abilities. More positive associations of families with their older members may then reshape attitudes and change prejudices.

Any new approach has limitations, pitfalls, and clinical challenges. The field is new and unsupported by a large body of professional literature. The practical application of integrated family models has not yet captured the attention of major researchers. Consequently, the model for a family-centered approach has evolved in the clinical realm, where its limitations, challenges, and pitfalls are readily sensed. The clinician, as Beatman (1967) said, must first deal with "unfinished business" between generations in order to facilitate structural as well as symptomatic changes in the family's potential as a treatment milieu.

The clinician or other helping professional must anticipate dealing with "unfinished business" between generations as well as planning for symptomatic relief of problems that emerge during the course of long-term treatment. Clinical problem areas in a family-centered approach include the family's tendency to deny or minimize symptoms, cure-seeking routines, ownership issues, overloading of roles, difficulties with accepting limited treatment objectives, and difficulties in maintaining continuity in relational patterns when the impaired member is placed out of the home.

This chapter reviews the promises and pitfalls of a family management model from a clinical perspective. It is by no means exhaustive, but it is offered to assist professional workers organize their own thinking in this challenging area. Despite some limitations, the value of a family management model as an integrator of intergenerational relationships far outweighs the current limitations.

IDENTIFYING SPECIFIC CHALLENGES IN FAMILY MANAGEMENT

The ability to cope effectively with a variety of stress is necessary to the quality of life. Families with impaired elderly must learn to live with some stress and strain. The challenge to the professional is one way of keeping the inevitable stressors from overwhelming the family's capacity to restore its own equilibrium. Stress responses occur at many levels of family functioning; they are an evitable feature of even normal family interliving. However, too much stress is presumed, though not proven, to accelerate the "aging process" itself by aggravating psychological, behavioral, and physical decline in later life. Since aging neurons may exhibit less capacity to adapt to stress, the older person may become less stress-resistive and consequently more vulnerable to family-related stress.

Family relational patterns often eventuate in stressful situations, particularly during later life because of the mismatch or lack of balance between care demands and the family's ability to respond without unreasonable cost to individual members. Optimal adjustment demands that individual members tolerate in some measure ongoing confusion, value conflict, and ambiguities.

Stress can be acute, beginning suddenly and terminating within a short time, or it can be chronic and continuous. Stress responses can vary from merely exciting to exhilarating to annoying to incapacitating, depending on how the family unit defines the events. One family might define the aging process in terms of harm, loss, and threats to family functioning; another family might perceive the process as an opportunity for growth, mastery, or gain.

Whether the family's response is one of denial, defensiveness, or depression, the emotions surrounding specific events are largely reactions to how actual, imagined or anticipated events are defined. The professionals should aid in redefinition of events if stress is overwhelming the family's adaptive response capacity. Given the view that the older member is more susceptible to stress in general, specific stress management techniques may become part of the overall treatment process.

According to Kalish and Collier (1981, pp. 219–213), acute stress or anxiety reactions appear to follow a general progressive track comprised of roughly five stages: (1) awareness, (2) initial reaction, (3) response, (4) outcomes, and (5) posttraumatic response. Awareness has to do with cognition that stressful events are about to happen. At this stage, the individual mobilizes resources for coping with what is about to happen. Prolonged anticipation in the *awareness* stage often proves to be more stressful than the anticipated event itself. Following awareness and mobilization, the individual expresses an overt or covert emotional response of acceptance or denial, anger or fear. In preparing for "fight or flight," the individual may experience an enhanced effectiveness in the *initial reaction* stage; however, confusion, numbness, reduced effectiveness of sensory and motor responses, restricted attention, memory failure, and "suspension of affective awareness" (Weiss & Payson, 1967) are more characteristic responses. The subsequent *response* may be resistance, culminating in exhaustion, which is some movement of the system toward regaining balance. If stress is prolonged or too intense, the *outcomes* involve seeking outside resources to help in reestablishing balance. Weiss and Payson (1967) describe the fifth stage as a posttraumatic response involving a reconstruction of the self and its relationships. Many symptoms presented to the clinicians, particularly psychosomatic complaints by one or more family members, have their origin in stress responses but should not be ignored or denied.

Chronic or prolonged stress follows a different pathway as families often develop adaptive and nonadaptive coping strategies for the exigencies of the aging process. The responses of these families have been characterized by Anderson (1981) as the "giving-up–given-up." Speer (1970) notes that these families use certain repetitive and enduring techniques for stress management and maintenance of balance.

Schmale and Engel (1967) first described the "giving-up–given-up" complex in their work with depressed individuals. Anderson (1981) then applied this conceptualization to family stress reaction patterns. The concept includes five psychological characteristics expressed in relational patterns: (1) feelings of helplessness and hopelessness, (2) a depreciated self-image, (3) a sense of lost gratification, (4) a sense of discontinuity, and (5) reactivation of past failures. These five attributes are reflected in the "giving-up" phase; the "given-up" phase, which may or may not follow, is marked by the apparent finality of loss. The consequences of the concept for the family are varied. The family may evolve new coping strategies or effect changes in environmental demands that restore balance. One or more members may become physically ill as a method of reducing the demands or one or more members may develop severe psychosocial disruptions that redefine the family's relationship to the external world. The aged and their families are in all probability highly susceptible to the giving-up–given-up complex.

The "giving-up" posture is reflected in feelings of helplessness in the face of the environmental demands and feelings of hopelessness in the face of the individual's ability to master the environmental demands. The self is viewed as less competent and less capable. Gratification or sources of reinforcement are lost or perceived to be lost, as crucial life roles defining status and relationships change.

The overwhelming present is viewed as significantly different from the past, and forecasts become more difficult to develop. Memories of past failures are reactivated; each successive loss, no matter how minor, is experienced as representative of all loss.

Anderson (1981) recommends restoration of a sense of control for families suffering from this complex. Learned helplessness is based on the assumption of no control. Families first must be helped to realize that they do have control over many aspects of psychological distress through a variety of therapeutic techniques. Second, the elderly must be reinvested with appropriate "power" to impact events surrounding them. Participatory decision making is one way to return power to those who have given up. Third, the real and perceived losses must be cast into terms of "operationalized mourning" that will allow for expression of grief. The family should be encouraged to express feelings surrounding the losses. Guilt, anger, resentment, remorse, blame, and ambivalence are natural and common grief reactions.

The highly stressed family and the "given-up" family pose particular limitations to the clinician using the family-centered approach because of stress contagion and negativism. The clinician must guard against participating in the family's reactions and must maintain objectivity. The "job description" and contracting approaches may help in identifying appropriate control areas for both professionals and families.

The process of conjoint problem solving demands professional commitment to ongoing appraisal of the effectiveness of interventions and readjustment when the interventions are not optimally effective. However, readjustments must not be too abrupt, and they must not undermine the progress that the family has made in accommodating physiological distress. Situations that require escalation of supportive resources or out-of-home placement to meet the care needs of impaired elderly must be approached with the same concern for family continuity as in-home services. When in-home support is not sufficient to maintain the integrity of the older person and the family system, out-of-home placement should be considered. The issue of maintaining family control and continuity even in case of relocation of the impaired member to other service delivery sites, such as senior apartment complexes, daycare centers, and nursing homes, is particularly challenging to the professional. Other difficulties inherent in a family-centered approach include the family's reluctance to seek treatment and the professional's reluctance to treat the disease and decline of older persons optimistically.

DENIAL: SYMPTOMS vs. HELP SEEKING

Families working with their older members are subject to a variety of attitudes, prejudices, and misunderstandings of the aging process and varying personal motivations that affect their sensitive and timely identification of problems. Negative attitudes, prejudices, and misunderstandings are unfortunately part of our socialization patterns. The popular images of older people are for the most part as senile, nonproductive, and deteriorating people. Hopefully, a clearer understanding of the aging process and exposures to healthy aging processes will shape more positive attitudes and eliminate prejudices for future generations. Meanwhile, older family members are affected by the misunderstandings of their families.

Personal motivations and commitments to problem solving vary among family members. Likewise, each family member including the older person has a vested interest in maintaining specific roles and relationships within the family structure. Role changes within families may proceed at different rates. Individuals may be relatively prepared for an expected role change or totally unprepared. Rates of individual role change do not necessarily synchronize. This presents major challenges in managing family problems, understanding multiple layers of family interaction, and clarifying individual motivations within the family. The true nature of roles and acceptance of the role responsibilities within the family structure may be apparent only after extensive evaluation of the family system. Families may resist this extensive evaluation in order to preserve the relative stability of individual roles.

Attitudes, prejudices, and misunderstandings may motivate family members to approach problem identification and solution in different ways. Family members may be highly invested in maintaining the status quo and may resist change. Evaluation by outsiders may represent a threat to the status quo. Furthermore, the subtle changes of their older members may be relatively easy to deny, minimize, or rationalize. Family members may not want to rock the boat for fear of losing status or role, prescriptions that may change the family system in unalterable ways. Families may be satisfied with the quality of the system as it is rather than invest in developmental progression or problem solutions. Clinicians sense this resistivity in directives from family members such as "don't do too much," "leave them in peace," or "just make them comfortable."

Family members may also see the evaluation process as a direct challenge to the family's effectiveness and indicative of their family's failures. They may attribute problem-solving failures to the older member's lack of cooperation, stubbornness, or willfulness. This leads to premature withdrawal from the problem.

Resistivity to timely and accurate evaluation of the problems of aging takes a variety of forms. Direct denial of problems is evident in the following case example. A 71-year-old male presented for evaluation and treatment of a long-term alcohol problem. Over the last several years he had been drinking constantly, with associated periods of depression. The patient's history included two major suicide attempts, which had been denied and ignored by the family.

The patient had jumped into a river during the winter with the intent of killing himself. He had to be removed forcibly. He had also attempted to hang himself from barn rafters, where he was cut down, suffering only rope burns to his neck. The family was apparently able to deny the alcohol abuse and depressive symptoms including overt suicide attempts until he started making inappropriate and irrational sexual comments about his wife in public. At that point, the family found help.

Another form of resistance to evaluation and treatment involves minimizing the problems. An 83-year-old male with clear evidence of dementia, an impaired gait, "bed sores," and major deterioration in functional capacity was maintained in his home by his wife and middle-aged son. The history of gradual intellectual decline, loss of speech function, and impaired gait had been minimized as "minor changes." The "bed sores" resulting from immobility were also ignored. He presented for evaluation to an acute care hospital only after suffering a mild stroke. The focal neurological finding of left-sided weakness resulting from the stroke could not be minimized by the family, and treatment was finally sought.

Another form of minimizing the problems of aging is clear in the following case example. A 69-year-old retired male with adult-onset diabetes and arteriosclerotic heart disease had difficulty adjusting to retirement. He had a two-year history of increasingly severe depressive features, including social withdrawal, apathy, decreased cognitive output, and a blunted depressed affect. The family minimized the severity of these symptoms and trusted the physician, who knew the patient well, to discover the difficulty and to intervene.

The pathology became more pronounced, and the family was unable to dismiss the old member's constant bed rest and minimal participation in daily activities. Finally, the family began to explore the history of symptoms with the patient's general physician. At that time, they learned that the behavior changes coincided with the physician's increased doses of valium nearly to an abusive level. The physician and patient had successfully hidden from the direct family scrutiny the amount and effects of the drug therapy. The physician in this case had reinforced the family's denial by his own secrecy and silence.

Other forms of resistivity to clinical intervention are more clearly rationalizations attributing problems to natural causes and normal aging. A 73-year-old widow successfully adjusted to the death of her husband and reestablished an active social life, involvement in the community, and adequate psychological adjustment. The neighbors and family over a period of a year, however, noticed a gradual change in her energy level, emotional resilience, and basic housekeeping and food preparation. Her previously immaculate house became messy, her kitchen disorganized, and her clothes disheveled. She repeatedly rationalized these changes with the explanation, "this is how it is when you grow older.'' The family, not wanting to usurp her autonomy and reduce her independence, accepted the rationalization. The patient then developed unstable angina and died rather suddenly of a massive heart attack. Change in function and behavior that the patient and family had rationalized as part of normal aging had in reality been progressive integrated arteriosclerotic heart disease.

DECLINE: MAINTENANCE vs. CURES

Acceptance of decline in physical and mental functioning is difficult at any age but is expecially poignant among older people: ''It's rough when you lose a little bit all the time.'' Failure to accept decline can be seen as an extension of denial. Although the older person admits to some difficulties, another level of denial surfaces as the older person struggles to accept the lack of possible cures. The reality of *irreversible* decline is vigorously denied. The emotional conflicts, frustrations, and resistances to maintenance interventions rather than curative interventions affect families, professionals, and older persons alike.

An older person's failure to accept decline is illustrated in the following case example. An 85-year-old female bitterly complained about the circulatory, structural, and skin changes of her legs. Her joints were enlarged and moderately deformed due to long-term arthritis, and her ankles were frequently edematous due to vascular insufficiency. Seeking cures, she saw a number of physicians. When mild diuretics, exercise, and analgesics were recommended for maintenance, she would aggressively confront the physicians, demanding a cure.

The typical response of a family to the decline of Alzheimer's disease is further illustrated in the family's resistance to decline in function. A 79-year-old man presented for evaluation with his family. The family gave a history of progressive, slow intellectual decline over the past three years. The symptoms of short-term memory deficit, disorientation to time and place, and inability to abstract information from the environment clearly pointed to a diagnosis of dementing disease. The family, however, had consulted three physicians who took the history, completed comprehensive evaluations, and diagnosed the disease as Alzheimer's. The realization of progressive and complete decline of the family member was overwhelming. The family appeared almost driven in urgent and desperate search for a different diagnosis and cure.

Even doctors have difficulty accepting irreversible decline. This is apparent in the following case. A 79-year-old male suffered a gradual onset of a mild gait instability characterized by a shuffle, difficulty pivoting quickly, and a slowed pace. His general physician, frustrated with the change, referred him to a rheumatologist, then a series of two independent neurologists for an extensive battery of tests with the result of no definite reversible pathology. Only then was the physician able to develop a maintenance plan for the problem.

DISEASE: MEDICAL SUPREMACIES vs. SHARED OWNERSHIP

Disease is a reality with increased age along with frustration and pain. Consequently, there are many personal, family, and professional conflicts, opinions, and struggles surrounding the disease process. The current medical model approaches disease from the perspective of diagnosis, treatment, and cure. The limitations of this acute medical care model are abundantly clear in the area of problem solution for the aged. Problems of aging directly challenge the utility of a model based on treatment and cure. However, the medical model is powerful and pervasive. Unfortunately, the lack of a clear process for sharing ownership of aging problems across disciplines and services represents a less popularly understood counterpart of this medical model supremacy. The supremacy of the medical model and lack of a sense of shared ownership represent a major pitfall in family management of aging problems.

The supremacy of the medical model is one of the main precipitants of battles over turfdom or territoriality between disciplines and service providers. Disease in aging is a reality. However, this reality also includes a different confidence and reliability of clinical diagnosis in the aged, a broad range of biological treatments, and an end result of change in the psychological and social function, *not* cure. In other words, the psychological and social results of diseases are equally as important as biological change. Attempts to blend professional skills from biological, psychological, and social areas are one way to accentuate power struggles.

Turfdom is popularly understood in a variety of ways. Frequently, turfdom refers to competition for financial resources and the battles of each discipline to justify its existence to capture increasingly limited resources. Turfdom also results from lack of role focus, clarity, or common stated goal. The biological goal of curing disease is quite different from the psychological goal of maximizing function or the social goal of maintaining supports. Opinions, priorities, and actions of different disciplines and service providers create issues of turfdom, which only serve to demoralize the family further.

The destructiveness of medical supremacy, lack of shared ownership, and turfdom is painfully clear in the following case examples. The supremacy of diagnosis is clear in the following cases. A 67-year-old divorced male presented for medication review. The primary reason for this review was to meet the requirements of the nursing home where he resided rather than identify, evaluate, or treat problems. His history included a chronic alcohol abuse pattern and a history of Wernicke-Korsakoff's psychosis four years prior to presentation for medication evaluation. Subsequent history included a two and one-half year hospitalization at a state mental hospital and a one and one-half year stay at the nursing home.

When evaluated for his "medication review," he displayed no evidence of confusion, memory impairment, or eye-movement abnormalities, yet medical management for four years had been based on this diagnosis. His functional capacity appeared intact; in fact, his social skills, organizational skills, and adequate cognitive function resulted in his election as president of the residents' council at the nursing home. Further exploration of his previous hospitalizations revealed no evidence of confusion, disorientation, or eye-movement abnormalities on admission despite the diagnosis of Wernicke-Korsakoff's psychosis. Neuropsychological testing to explore the specifics of his cognitive function at that time was not accomplished. Clearly, the power of a diagnostic label had directed his life for the past four years. The initial diagnosis upon review was questionable and not clearly documented. Furthermore, it had not been reevaluated but accepted by service providers as he was passed along the continuum.

An 83-year-old female was admitted for comprehensive evaluation of her left hip. Results of examination and X-rays revealed a hip fracture, which was treated surgically and followed by a rehabilitation program. When she was walking successfully, she was released from treatment. With her walker, she returned to her trailer, where her entryway steps were made of crumbling concrete blocks. The steps had no rail. She refused to ask for help in negotiating these steps; once she was in her trailer, she stayed there, unnecessarily captive in her own house. Her hip had been treated and was healed, but her psychosocial competencies had been eroded.

The supremacy of the disease concept and failure to see beyond the disease to functional change is clear in the following case. A 71-year-old man presented with his wife for evaluation of a diagnosis of Alzheimer's disease made several years earlier. He had received no medical attention in the last 10 years. His wife had managed his personal care, his business, his decision making, and every major function of his life. She expected him to be confused, cognitively impaired, and helpless because of the diagnosis and information that the initial evaluating physician had shared with her. Review of the onset of his problem revealed that a gradual visual loss and mild confusion had followed a head injury as a result of a car accident. The mild confusion interfered with his vocational function, and he was released from an active work responsibility. Agitation had been briefly controlled with major tranquilizers and a state hospital placement. The patient's wife then became frustrated with his treatment and returned him to their home, where she managed his care without medication or support. When evaluated, he was pleasant, cooperative, and extremely dependent on his wife. Only mild memory deficits could be detected; the major dysfunctions appeared to be depression, social withdrawal, and sensory deprivation. A misdiagnosis of Alzheimer's disease had supported his major functional impairment despite only minor deficits for over 12 years.

There is a variety of popular reactions against the supremacy of the medical model. The medical model needs to be challenged; however, the antagonism and aggression of these reactions must be tempered with a humanistic concern for the people affected. A spirit of shared ownership of problems is the most reasonable course for both families and professionals.

The antimedical posture can also be destructive. This is clear in the following case. An 81-year-old widow had recently moved across country to live closer to her only family member, a son. She had made this decision with the counsel of her son after care of her house and business affairs had become too difficult. She had a long history of mild paranoid symptoms and subsequent difficulties with her immediate neighbors as well as difficulties enlisting supportive help. She trusted her son, though in recent years they had not been close. However, she chose to move near her son and his family.

She presented for psychiatric evaluation when the son became increasingly concerned about repeated short-term memory failure and periods of confusion. After initial evaluation, discussion with the patient's general physician, and subsequent workup, a diagnosis of early Alzheimer's disease was made. Appropriate intervention appeared to be guardianship appointment and placement in a semistructured retirement center. This placement was accomplished; however, staff at this facility immediately aligned with the patient, told her she was completely healthy after a brief screening interview by a social worker, and assisted the patient in securing an attorney, a realtor, and a different physician. This reaction against the medical opinion resulted in a long, painful guardianship appointment, alienation of the patient from rehabilitation programs, and bad feelings toward the son and his family. The retirement center staff was totally unreceptive to discussing the problems and reacted as if the physician and family had abused the patient. The psychological destructiveness of their behavior was abundantly clear in the subsequent marginal adjustment of the patient.

Lack of a sense of shared ownership and responsibility is frighteningly evident in the following case. Another extremely painful detail of this case includes a series of problems and system intervention failures. Repeated failures of individual systems to share ownership of problems resulted in great psychological pain to the individual. A 79-year-old widow living in her home called several nursing homes to inquire about available services. She sounded mildly confused and upset over the phone, and the nursing home's social worker appropriately referred her to the Office on Aging supportive services. The information and referral worker began a systematic screening in the woman's home, where she found poor housekeeping, disorganization, and evidence of poor personal care including inadequate meals. Communication with the woman was complicated by her hearing impairment, major defensiveness, poor self-esteem, and personal feeling of failure when help was offered.

Before appropriate referrals and support services could be instituted, the Office on Aging supervisor advised the intake worker to let the woman care for herself and not foster dependence (mistake 1). The woman then fell victim to major financial exploitation when a community person befriended her, sold her house illegally (mistake 2), and kept the money. She then surfaced at a local nursing home, where her physician had admitted her following superficial examination, subsequent diagnosis of severe depression, and no referral for treatment (mistake 3).

Her persistent hopelessness, helplessness, depression, and report of being "taken" to the nursing home prompted nursing home staff to request a psychiatric evaluation. During a month of individual work, it became apparent that she suffered from mild cognitive impairment and had been the victim of financial exploitation. At that point, the case was referred to the Office on Aging ombudsman, who facilitated a complete and thorough legal evaluation. The case attracted media attention early in the process; a television investigative reporter interviewed the woman and aired the coverage prematurely (mistake 4). When the case went to court, the case was dismissed (mistake 5). Meanwhile, the woman had lived in the nursing home on welfare, disinterested in activities, socially withdrawn and uncommunicative.

This series of system mistakes, not one system's mistake but several interrelated mistakes, resulted in two years of psychological pain and discomfort for the woman. The failure of sensing shared responsibility and ownership of the woman's problems itself became a secondary problem in the aging process.

DEATH: QUALITY OF LIFE

Death as the final stage in life and dying as the final process are important issues for older individuals and their families. Older people think and talk about death more frequently and are generally less fearful of death than younger people (Feifel & Branscomb, 1973). Kalish and Reynolds (1976) point out that older people may be more accepting of the fact of death due to a sense of diminished social value, a sense of completeness about life, and socialization to their own death through experience with the death of spouse and peers. Lindemann (1944) discusses the ability to integrate one's death in relationship to the capacity to tolerate loss or the process of mourning. He defines the completion of this process and integration into the current state of being in the stages of denial, depression, and subsequent readjustment.

Further exploration of factors that influence the acceptance of death have resulted in little specific information relative to the aging individual. Kalish (1976) points out that older people appear to fear prolonged illness, dependency, and pain more than death itself. There appears to be no greater concern about death among the chronically ill than among healthy population. However, the terminally ill revealed much greater anxiety and depression than the chronically ill or healthy population (Feifel & Branscomb, 1973). It is clear from other research that the particular illness causing death has a profound influence on how death is perceived and handled.

The hospice concept has developed in response to the need for support of the terminally ill to counter the major fear of dying alone and in pain. In medieval Europe, the hospice represented a shelter for travelers on difficult journeys. In modern times, hospice has come to mean a program for care of dying patients and support for their families. The hospice idea represents a philosophy of care rather than a place and is accomplished in a variety of locations including hospital-based, community-based, or home-based programs. Care is delivered by a physician-directed interdisciplinary team with 24-hour a day care available. The orientation of hospice care is to provide compassionate care and pain relief during the dying process rather than rehabilitation or discharge planning. Family involvement is an integral part of the concept. Bereavement counseling is a follow-up component of hospice care. There are approximately 300 hospices across the United States, with a national hospice organization setting standards and coordinating information exchange.

The commitment and effectiveness of hospice care are revealed by the following case example. A 69-year-old woman developed metastatic breast cancer three years after a radical mastectomy and radiation treatment. She had made the initial adjustment after surgery, returning to active involvement in civic and volunteer groups within the community. However, the psychological stress of readjustment was evident as she began to lose physical energy and psychological stamina with the spreading metastasis. She was referred to hospice care, suffering from major depression, social withdrawal, and noncompliance with routine management of pain.

The hospice worker was able to provide a supportive relationship for the patient outside her family. Her noncompliance with pain medications was explored. She had observed her father die an early death from alcoholism and feared use of pain medications herself, due to a perceived addictive potential. The hospice worker arranged nursing education about pain management; with support she was able to commit to a quality of life and pain control in her terminal stage. She was able to reengage in some civic activities on a more limited basis. The appetite disturbance was managed through preparation of favorite foods by neighbors and friends. She continued active involvement with her family at home until a respiratory infection and further physical deterioration required admission to the hospital component of the hospice program. She died in the hospital. Ongoing family education and support prior to death had helped prepare the family for the loss. The hospice worker continued follow-up visits with the patient's husband through the first year after her death.

AVOIDING PROFESSIONAL OVERLOAD

The case examples demonstrate that demands made on families in a family-centered treatment approach to the psychological distress of aging are diverse and complex. The demands made on the health care professional are equally diverse and complex. Both parties may suffer from conflicts and role overload if their general responsibilities are not circumscribed from the onset of treatment. The role of the family has been described throughout this text. The role of the clinician or other professional must also be carefully delineated if shared ownership of treatment outcomes is to be realized effectively. The professional must become like a broker, negotiating the supply/demand attitudes that permeate care services. The professional must coordinate those services once negotiated, monitor the goodness-of-fit of demands with resources, and evaluate future care planning needs for individual family members, the family as a unit, and the impaired member. This coordination must be effected against a backdrop of family resistivity, fragmented community-based services, and a professional mentality that fails to perceive the family as the actual client/patient in treatment objectives for impaired elderly. Referral processes, reimbursement patterns, and most required record keeping for serving, further fragment the treatment approaches and must be creatively circumvented by the clinician. Feelings of anger, grief, helplessness, hopelessness, and ambivalence by both professionals and families at times divide and obscure treatment aims.

It is often difficult for the professionals to maintain role integrity in the face of such diverse and intense response demands. Controlled distancing from problematic family relationships and from the pathology of distressed members is often necessary. Therefore, it is important that the professional develop a "job description" at the onset of treatment. This case-by-case job description should detail who will do what for whom, under what circumstances, and how long. It must be developed with reference to the presenting need of the impaired member and with reference to the family structural preference for configuration, coordination, and closure (see Chapter 4). Since the family system is to be used as a treatment milieu, the professional must appraise existing resources and identify additional resources that may be used to amplify treatment strategies.

Reifler and Eisdorfer (1980) studied the use of psychiatric outpatient clinics by families with impaired elderly. They found that at the time of the first visit the family had been experiencing problems for a year or more. The actual visits usually had varied precipitants, but in most cases family members had begun contemplation of out-of-home placement or guardianship for the older person. The families were beset with guilt, confused about their responsibilities, and uncertain as to the best course of action.

Treatment then must deal with goals of symptomatic relief as well as more significant longer-term goals of structural changes, while avoiding overload of professionals and families. An understanding of these processes aids the professional in writing a case-specific job description.

There are several goals in family-centered intervention such as decreased dependencies and vulnerability of the impaired older person through increased functional capacities; increased predictability and stability of the family as a treatment milieu; decreased anxiety and stress surrounding caretaking; increased knowledge about normal and atypical care demands and subsequent service needs; and increased skills and confidence in family members' abilities to manage current and future problems associated with psychological distress of aging. In order to be realized, these goals should be operationalized step-by-step so that the professional's job description consists of at least five broad phases of intervention: (1) connecting, (2) mobilizing, (3) contracting, (4) evaluating, and (5) feedback. Data for decision making about these phases are obtained from the assessment process described in Chapter 3. Minuchin (1974) observes that a clinician must necessarily become a part of the family system before attempting to change the system. Basic to connecting with families is a demonstrated respect for boundaries. The assessment of family attributes may aid the clinician in connecting with families' perspectives of the problem; the older person's past, current, and future role in the family; past experiences with similar problems; how other family members, besides the primary informant or caretaker, feel about the problem; and what problem solutions have been tried, succeeded, or disallowed.

For example, if one member favors an all-or-none out-of-home placement solution and other members are seriously opposed, the clinician must attempt to understand, process, and empathize with both views. Connecting must occur, but it must be done with emotional integrity and controlled distancing; otherwise the clinician becomes a participatory member in whatever pathology exists. The clinician should take special care to delineate his or her role even in the connecting phase in order to provide an initial structure to the families' problem-solving strategies. Families who have either highly disengaged or highly enmeshed relational patterns are difficult for the professional to connect. Miller (1981) notes that disengaged families are relatively emotional isolates and interdependent; enmeshed families are so interdependent that members lack identity and autonomy. Fortunately, most families fall somewhere between the extremes of disengaged and enmeshed so that the clinician can connect without special strategies. Both extremes in family relational patterns—disengaged and enmeshed—may be difficult to mobilize.

The mobilization of family strengths requires a careful appraisal of the impaired person's needs and the family's actual ability to respond. Usually it is most helpful if the professional emphasizes the performance of specific, concrete treatment tasks that will contribute to the overall treatment process and aims. From the identification of specific tasks and specific assignments for family members, a clinician should then begin the process of treatment contracting. In contracting, "a mutual agreement about the goals, content, length, rules and methods of therapy is formally established" (Anderson, Hogarty, & Reiss, 1981, p. 83). The content of the contract should include the problem formulation statements resulting from the assessment process (see Chapter 3) as well as the results of alternative community resource identification if appropriate (see Chapter 6). Goal statements should contain both short-term and long-term aims, but major changes should be avoided in early stages of treatment. Contracting avoids a diffusion of treatment energies and subsequent ambiguities concerning treatment outcomes. The time framing of contracts, objectifying conjoint treatment activities, and establishing criteria or measurement of treatment outcomes avoid added stress and provide clear markers of treatment gains. The contract should be written, be signed by all members, and indicate review dates. A measurable device, or how one will know when a goal is realized, should also be built into the family contract.

Reifler and Eisdorfer (1980) found that while families often generate realistic overt treatment goals, they have an unrealistic covert expectation that the professional will provide a cure for the relative's problem. In view of this, the contract should be limited to three or four issues, with the flexibility to add more as they occur over the course of therapy. Goals for major structural or separation changes should be avoided in the early stages. Family complaints, however, should be translated into specific, clear, and attainable goal statements in the initial contract with the thought that as the family acquires new skills and information, the goals will change. Goal statements then help determine role statements.

Family life education or other knowledge needs also may be a part of the initial or subsequent contracts, especially if families are operating from an inaccurate or limited knowledge base. Usually, information about the psychological distress and suggestions for management and treatment including medications should be part of information sharing. Interpersonal stresses and individual vulnerability should be reviewed.

Before contracts are finalized, many families respond to distress in aging as if it were a short-term acute illness centering too much family responsiveness around "the illness." Over time this type of coping depletes the family's energy reserve and makes long-term care planning difficult. Consequently, ongoing maintenance management goals are emphasized along with short-term strategies for change.

Evaluation and feedback are critical phases in family-centered approaches that are too often minimized. Frequent review sessions should be conducted within the context of family conferences in order to identify accomplishments, reinforce morale, and anticipate emergent problem areas. Evaluation should be built into the contract itself in order to determine if the goals are realistic and if the change or maintenance strategies are working. If the contract is not working or not working very well after a reasonable trial, then new goals should be identified. Structured problem-solving methods often help the family review its own efforts and prevent false ownership of the problems by the clinician. If the treatment contract is not working, Falloon, Boyd, McGill, Strang, and Moss (1981) recommend that the following steps of structured problem solving should be utilized: (1) identify the specific problem area; (2) list alternative solutions/strategies; (3) discuss pros and cons, advantages and disadvantages; (4) choose a best-fit solution; (5) plan how to implement the solution; and (6) continue to review efforts.

This type of approach to initial treatment failures successfully reduces the level of tension, refocuses energies, and avoids falsely blaming or scapegoating the clinician or the service system. Feedback loops must be built into family-centered management in order to acknowledge goal attainment, avoid diffuse reactions, and prevent off-target agendas from infiltrating treatment planning efforts. The family-based assessment approach discussed in Chapter 3 can be used along with contract criteria to establish baselines of impaired performance. Reassessment then provides multiple measures of change or maintenance, identifies gaps in treatment efforts, and prescribes subsequent needed activities. Careful record keeping by families and professionals alike assures that a viable evaluation and feedback mechanism operates throughout the treatment.

In addition to the complexity of the presenting problem, other sources of overload are inherent in a family-centered approach. The organization of data and record keeping for multiple problems is difficult. In dealing with life spans, the amount of information relevant to the problem is often staggering, as well as the pervasiveness of the problem. Existing services are limited and fragmented, with rigid entitlement and admission criteria. Securing appropriate service is its own challenge to the humanistic professional. Lastly, the helping professional is limited in the quantity and quality of responsibilities that one individual can assume for assessment, treatment, conjoint case management, advocacy, and family and community education.

Stress in this model, then, can be traced to the ambiguities of outcomes in treatment plans, unclear cause-and-effect relationships in treating the impaired elderly and their families, and an inability to control multiple treatment variables. The results of professional role overload are manifested in a number of ways: loss of treatment objectivity, withdrawal or disengagement from treatment processes, and depression, cynicism, and pervasive pessimism concerning outcomes. The helping professional must guard against overload and realize that when family-centered approaches work, the credit for success is shared. When the approach fails, usually the family holds the professional responsible or professionals hold themselves responsible. If the recommended multidisciplinary team approach is utilized, then individual overload is somewhat minimized; however, the team as a whole is as susceptible to inherent pitfalls as individual professionals.

MAINTAINING FAMILY CONTINUITY IN ALTERNATIVE PLACEMENTS

One of the most serious potential limitations inherent in a family-centered approach is professional or family resistance to seeking more specialized long-term care services if provision of those services involves alternative placement of the impaired member. Families may be unrealistic in assuming all caretaking responsibilities or attempting to maintain the older person in their own or another member's home at an unreasonable cost to all.

The goal of long-term care is to improve, modify, and maintain the optimum level of function (Brody & Masciocchi, 1980). As the care needs of the impaired elderly change, the family should be encouraged to seek alternative placements to amplify their own caretaking resources. The alternatives are typically described as a collection of services existing along a care continuum with long-term care facilities and nursing homes at one end of the spectrum, in-home support at the other end, and many community-based services in the middle. There has been a tendency to describe this spectrum as extending along a dimension of restrictiveness. Gurland, Bennett, and Wilder (1981) recommend that the individual's needs match the services delivered along this continuum.

Families may decide, for a variety of reasons, that a higher level of care is needed; however, it appears that families lack a decision-making model for determination of appropriate alternatives especially when confronted with a crisis or conflict in caretaking (York & Calsyn, 1977). Families typically choose an all-or-none resolution resulting in nursing home placement. York and Calsyn (1977) report that the families in their study were not very systematic or sophisticated in their search for a nursing home. Availability of a bed and geographical location were the principal reasons given by families for the choice.

Linn and Gurel (1969) report a similar finding that the quality of meals at the nursing home was a significant factor in the families' selection of a particular site. Physicians and social workers were listed as important factors in the choice of a home for elderly who were hospitalized prior to the nursing home placement. The choice of placement most often is not guided by an assessment of the quality of care or by the involvement of the elderly patient in the decision making.

It appears that families should be supplied with a decision-making model relative to choices along a continuum and with a strategy for selecting a long-term facility if that is the preferred choice. A decision-making model relative to care needs of the impaired elderly should address these three broad issues: (1) determination of actual need based on a comprehensive assessment of functional capacity in relationship to current living environments; (2) identification and determination of available short-term and long-term service options relative to the intensity of the care demand and the appropriate service delivery location; and (3) determination and evaluation of outcomes of the utilization of alternatives in terms of the goals of short- and long-term care. The questions that a family must consider are: (1) What does the impaired person need in order to increase, maintain, or modify functional capacity? (2) Where can this service be delivered? (3) Does this service and service location meet the goals of long-term care or is the person getting what he or she needs in order to function in an optimal fashion?

Outcome measures of service alternatives are scarce for a number of practical and methodological reasons (Gurland, Bennett, & Wilder, 1981). The institutional industry has proliferated largely because of federal and state funding patterns, not because of careful evaluation of outcomes. Within the past two decades, nearly 1 million beds distributed among some 20,000 institutions have been established generally without regard to careful evaluation of the impact (Butler, 1975). Mace and Rabins (1981) recommend that a family considering out-of-home placement first investigate all funding options, not just the more obvious one; secure an adequate assessment/evaluation to determine the level of care needed; locate and evaluate the potential service delivery sites; and develop a placement plan that takes into account the adjustment needs of the family as well as the impaired individual. Mace and Rabins (1981) offer an excellent checklist for families considering nursing home placement that would be of considerable help (pp. 210–211).

Generally, families should consider three important dimensions in choosing a nursing home: (1) the physical facility, (2) the people who operate and inhabit the facility, and (3) the anticipated impact of the placement on the older person's sense of self, competence, and role within the family. The building should be evaluated in terms of its availability of beds; geographical proximity to family; cleanliness and overall maintenance; safety; eating, sleeping, and activity areas; balance of social spaces with private use space, quiet areas, and social activity areas; availability of services such as beauty/barber shops, transportation, and libraries; and accessibility to surrounding community services.

The attitude of the staff toward the aged and the provision of care should be evaluated along with the availability of specialized professional services such as medical and psychiatric consultation and rehabilitation experts. Separation of care levels, staff turnover rates, staff development and training programs, and activity programs, both in-house and community-based, for different levels are important considerations. The staff ratio for different levels of care needs should also be assessed whenever possible.

The family must attempt to anticipate and plan for the impact of the placement in meeting the psychosocial as well as physical needs of older persons. Bengston (1973, p. 25) observes that the psychosocial needs of the elderly regardless of context include a need for maintaining "identity," maintaining "connectedness" with important relationships, and maintaining "affectance," which means having some sort of influence over or being able to "affect" the environment.

Families must scrutinize the alternative placement with reference to the organization's sensitivity to the older person's and the family's need to maintain identity, connectedness, and affectance. For example, families should ask, Do patients wear their own clothes and have their own furnishings? Are family visits encouraged? Is separate space provided for family visiting? Are any activities designed to include family members? Is every attempt made to keep the older person connected? Are the patients encouraged to participate in some of the program decisions? Is there a patient council? How can the older person change some routine or activity? How does the administration handle patient or family complaints? Is there any formal mechanism for affecting the environment?

Once an older person has been placed out of the home or moved to more specialized services, special steps must be taken to ensure the continuity of relational patterns. York and Calsyn (1977) found that, on the whole, families continue to visit and be concerned about the welfare of older members. However, their data also reveal that families need help in making their visits more productive. The great majority of families surveyed also reported that they would take part in any type of educational program that would make them more knowledgeable about the care of the older member. Clearly then, families should be helped in understanding how to visit their relatives and how to have their relatives visit them. Since families report the greatest difficulty in coping with mental deterioration and mood and memory disturbances, specific training should be offered for dealing with organic brain syndromes (senility) and related changes in behavior.

The Philadelphia Geriatric Center developed a booklet for families entitled "Visiting Your Relations" (Brody, 1977). In this booklet, the author stressed two major themes: (1) what to talk about, and (2) what to do together. Specifically it is suggested that family members encourage reminiscing, refrain from too much unsolicited advising, share family happenings, include friends or roommates in conversation, empathize with distressed feelings, and sympathize with the older person's frustrations. In terms of joint activities, it is recommended that family members do things with their relatives that they may have done in the past or things that they know might be very important to their older relatives. They may bring newspapers or magazines to be read and discussed; play games such as cards and dominoes; participate in decorating the patient's room; help with personal grooming choices; assist with letter writing; bring others to visit; bring pets if permissible; visit other areas of the facility; and take the relative for an outing.

Families usually wish to have the older person home for special events and holidays. Prior counseling of families and careful planning can ensure more successful and more frequent home visits.

The following set of ideas has been useful in helping families deal with home visits of older members with major cognitive impairments. The first question that should be answered is, Should the older relative visit? If the relative doesn't habitually visit at other times of the year, maybe intense holidays like Thanksgiving or Christmas aren't the best time to try. Instead of feeling guilty, the family might make plans for visiting during less stimulating holidays, e.g., Easter, Mother's Day, or Memorial Day; plan visits tied to "family" holidays like birthdays, anniversaries, clan gatherings, etc.; or plan to visit the older impaired person successfully where he or she is for the holiday.

Regardless of the options selected, families should be aware of the potential problems and plan for them. Generally, families have exceptionally high expectations for the holiday seasons—the magic cure of the holiday spirit. Family memories of their older members during happier, healthier holidays may overwhelm the family of the impaired and activate denial of problems, decline, and change as well as other deep emotions. Unrealistic expectations, stress, and generally increased energy demands often result in a holiday-disaster syndrome.

If an older person is to visit, the family should keep the following three guidelines in mind. First, there are problems with memory loss; the older impaired person is experiencing some memory losses. The excitement and information overload of the holiday may further influence the memory of impaired elderly. Avoid directly challenging the memory loss. Testing the limits of memory deficits doesn't make them go away but does set into motion a spiral of failure and anxiety. Support the older person's memory losses by giving him or her information, maybe showing photographs of family and friends who also will be visiting and preparing him or her in advance with concrete reminders.

Anticipate the problems with recognizing faces and associating faces with names. Supply them whenever possible. Be aware of delays in processing information. It takes an older person longer to respond; when talking with the older person, stay with a subject rather than quickly switching subjects. The older person can't follow as fast. Also the older person may have trouble understanding because of visual and hearing problems. The family should compensate by speaking clearly, at the right volume, one at a time, and should make sure that the older person understands. Use familiar items and familiar people to stimulate the memory. Provide necessary feeling bridges between the past and present. Help the older person associate the present—this holiday—with past holidays.

The second major problem area is confusion or the disorientation of impaired older persons. The family can help with this by providing simple direction or orientation to time, place, and person. For example, "Today is Christmas eve. Mary and George are coming to dinner tonight. It is now breakfast time but we have a lot of cooking to do." Simplify the environment and make it safe where possible, label the older person's bathroom or sleeping area, choose conversational topics that the older person not only knows but will be motivated to discuss—use familiar objects to provide stimuli.

Check with the nursing home if appropriate and get a schedule of normal activities including medication schedules. Don't expect the older person to know; in the excitement he or she may become even more confused.

Pace the social demands to allow for rest periods and stability zones. Remember that the whole visit might be overstimulating as well as overwhelming.

The last major problem area concerns feelings. The conversation and feelings of the older impaired person might be hard to follow because of the memory losses and disorientation. Sit back; relax; try to interpret the overall feeling, content, or theme; respond to that—don't deny the feelings such as "this might be our last holiday." Recognize and accept the need for an older person to prepare for death and possible incapacitation. Emphasize feelings; don't try to do therapy but joke, sing, laugh, and take in the feelings; don't insist that the older person feel differently. Go with the flow but avoid unnecessary upsets.

Don't give gifts from guilt. Look over the situation; select something useful, edible, or just plain enjoyable. Think about the past as well as what is presently valued by the older person.

Family education concerning problems in memory, mood, and behavior should be an ongoing process and should continue even after alternative placement of the older member. Continuity of care and continuity of relating are probably best secured through the family's active participation in development, implementation, and evaluation of nursing home care plans. Families can request to be included as part of the treatment team in ongoing maintenance plans; families should insist on being included in any change of care plans including any medication and activity changes. Families will assert more influence in the treatment of older members as their own knowledge base is expanded through the family-centered approach.

OTHER CONSIDERATIONS IN FAMILY CONTINUITY

The issues of competency, guardianship and conservatorship, and preservation of income often disrupt family care plans. The spouse or family caretaker may become ill, incapacitated, or even die. In chronic illnesses, it is important to plan along with the family for preservation of income and continued financing for provision of appropriate care services. Financial and legal issues that arise should be reviewed thoroughly with an attorney.

The questions of incompetence and guardianship are highly individual issues and should be considered on a case-by-case basis. While the authority to establish an individual's incompetence and subsequent guardianship is vested in the judiciary, the family must be able to participate appropriately if continuity is to be maintained. Different states provide for minimally restrictive levels of guardianship for impaired individuals such as voluntary guardianship or conservatorship. Once an individual is deemed incompetent, he or she becomes a "ward" and is not expected to participate in decisions affecting care and finances (Hyland, 1980). The following categories of legal actions that families can take should be considered with reference to legal statutes for the state of legal residency, since state laws vary with respect to these issues.

The degree of dysfunction should be carefully thought through, and the individual's rights should not be usurped unnecessarily. An impaired elderly may not be able to balance a checkbook but be competent and able to make a will assigning power of attorney to an adult child, close friend, or spouse. The power of attorney gives the invested individual authority to manage certain financial transactions and make other specified decisions in granting the individual's best interests. A *conservatorship* or *guardian of property* requires a formal judicial hearing to determine an individual's competency. As a result of the petition, a judge may appoint a legal guardian to act for the person in only financial matters or appoint a *guardianship of person,* a more complex and encompassing responsibility, which involves decisions related to assessment and treatment.

Any of these procedures affects the individual's rights and disrupts family role patterns. However, it may be equally important to families' continuity of care to protect an impaired member's rights by formalizing certain anticipated transactions, particularly financial ones. In cases of dementing illness, it is important to involve the individual and family in joint planning to preserve income and safeguard basic rights as early as possible so that the individual can understand and act on his or her own behalf. Early involvement enables families to develop anticipatory plans free from feelings of guilt or recrimination as alternative placements are sought.

REFERENCES

Anderson, C.M., Hogarty, G., & Reiss, D.J. The psychoeducational family treatment of schizophrenia. In M.J. Goldstein (Ed.), *New directions for mental health services: New developments in interventions with families of schizophrenics.* San Francisco: Jossey-Bass, 1981.

Anderson, J.T. The family that gives up. In G. Getty and W. Humphrey (Eds.), *Understanding the family: Stress and change in American family life.* New York: Appleton-Century-Crofts, 1981.

Beatman, F.L. Intergenerational aspects of family therapy. In N.W. Ackerman (Ed.), *Expanding theory and practice in family therapy.* New York: Family Service Association of America, 1967.

Bengston, V.L. The institutionalized aged and their social needs. In *Psychosocial needs of the aged: Selected papers.* Los Angeles: University of Southern California, The Ethel Percy Andrus Gerontology Center, 1973. (Monograph)

Brody, E.M. Visiting your relatives at the Philadelphia Geriatric Center: A note to family and friends of our residents. In E.M. Brody (Ed.), *Long-term care of older people: A practical guide.* New York: Human Sciences Press, 1977.

Brody, S.J., & Masciocchi, C. Data for long-term care planning by health systems agencies. *American Journal of Public Health,* 1980, *70* (11), 1194–1198.

Butler, R. *Why survive: On growing old in America.* New York: Harper and Row, 1975.

Falloon, R.H., Boyd, J.L., McGill, C.W., Strang, J.S., & Moss, H.B. Family management training in the community care of schizophrenia. In M.J. Goldstein (Ed.), *New directions for mental health services: New developments in interventions with families of schizophrenics.* San Francisco: Jossey-Bass, 1981.

Feifel, H., & Branscomb, A.B. Who's afraid of death? *Journal of Abnormal Psychology,* 1973, *81,* 282–288.

Gurland, B., Bennett, R., & Wilder, D. Reevaluating the place of evaluation in planning for alternatives to institutional care for the elderly. *Journal of Social Issues,* 1981, *37* (3), 51–70.

Hyland, D.J. The legal side: Incompetence and guardianship. *American Journal of Nursing,* October 1980, 1163–1164.

Kalish, R.A. Death and dying in a social context. In R.H. Binstock and E. Shanas (Eds.), *Handbook of aging and the social sciences.* New York: D. Van Nostrand, 1976.

Kalish, R.A., & Collier, K.W. *Exploring human values.* Monterey, Calif.: Brooks/Cole, 1981.

Kalish, R.A., & Reynolds, D.K. *Death and ethnicity: A psychocultural study.* Los Angeles: University of Southern California Press, 1976.

Lindemann, E. Symptomatology and management of acute grief. *American Journal of Psychiatry,* 1944, *101,* 141–148.

Linn, M.W., & Gurel, L. Initial reactions to nursing home placement. *Journal of American Geriatrics Society,* 1969, *17,* 219–223.

Mace, N.L., & Rabins, P.V. *The 36-hour day: A family guide to caring for persons with Alzheimer's disease, related dementing illnesses and memory loss in later life.* Baltimore: The Johns Hopkins University Press, 1981.

Miller, J.R. Family support of the elderly. *Family and Community Health,* 1981, *3* (4), 39–49.

Minuchin, S. Structural family therapy. In S. Arieti (Ed.), *American handbook of psychiatry* (Vol. 2). New York: Basic Books, 1974.

Reifler, B.V., & Eisdorfer, C. A clinic for the impaired elderly and their families. *American Journal of Psychiatry,* 1980, *137* (11), 1399–1403.

Schmale, A., and Engel, G. The giving up-given up complex. *Archives of General Psychiatry,* 1967, *17,* 134–145.

Speer, D. Family systems: Morphostasis and morphogenesis, or is homeostatis enough? *Family Process,* 1970, *9,* 259–278.

Weiss, R.J., & Payson, H.E. Gross stress reaction: I. In A.M. Freedman and H.I. Kaplan (Eds.), *Comprehensive textbook of psychiatry.* Baltimore: Williams and Wilkins, 1967.

York, J.L., & Calsyn, R.J. Family involvement in nursing homes. *Gerontologist,* 1977, *17,* 500–505.

Chapter 8

Wellness and Maintenance of Mental Health

The maintenance of mental health and prevention of the psychological distresses associated with aging demand a clear understanding of the developmental tasks of late life. Popular views of the tasks of later life are often superficial and limited. Perceived outcomes of healthy aging are assumed to include development of wisdom, adjustment to life change, and survival of numerous life experiences. Further elaboration of these issues rarely demystifies the aging process for the general public and usually doesn't contribute to greater understanding of aged persons. The mental health of older people becomes subject to a variety of myths and stereotypes. The older individual is faced with the challenge of completing developmental tasks of personality integration in an environment that is not conducive to successful completion (Verwoerdt, 1981).

The maintenance of an older individual's mental health can be understood by sensitive observation and facilitation of his or her personality integration. Erikson (1959) defines this integration as a positive and genuine acceptance of choices regarding lifelong environmental demands and relational patterns. Verwoerdt (1981) defines this task as the final integration of one's current self and all past selves. Weinberg (1979) defines the process as acceptance of one's legend or personal biography as valuable, worthwhile, and complete.

Another approach to understanding and facilitating these later-life tasks involves support of the process skills involved: identity, relating, and control. The older individual must actively pursue the definition and redefinition of self across time. This self-definition or identity must include a clear understanding of the biophysical self, including physical health, physical maintenance, and physical limitations; a clear understanding of the psychological self or inner life of subjective experience and personal adaptations; and a clear understanding of the social self in family relationship roles such as grandparenting and changes in work roles and leisure time. The interactive nature of these three areas of self-definition is abundantly clear. Good health alone is not a complete answer

Figure 8-1 Interaction of Identity, Relating, and Control in Maintenance of Mental Health

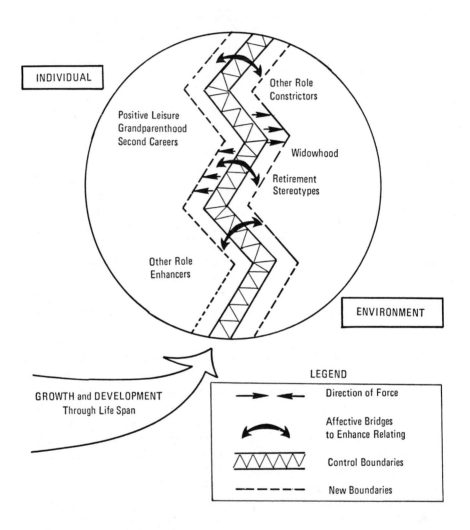

to good mental health. Complete independence of the inner self is not conducive to good mental health. The recluse living alone with his or her cats is rarely viewed as psychosocially competent. Social relationships in the absence of physical health and psychological adjustments do not create a sense of completeness for the social butterfly.

This complex definition of self or identity interacts in a reciprocal fashion with environmental demands of a person's relating or connection to environmental figures. The intricacies of lifelong relationships must be reviewed in later life and integrated for good mental health. The individual self does not define his or her identity in a void but rather in terms of the cognitive and affective bonds established in experienced relationships along the life course. The widow or widower must redefine self and restructure relationships after death of a spouse. Likewise, the newly retired individual must redefine self in relationship to a different environment of leisure and fewer structured contacts with coworkers.

The complex interaction of individual identity and relationship to environment is under the control of the individual. Ego function or control mechanisms regulate the boundaries of self and fine tune the balance between identity directed toward the environment or identity directed inward. Control mechanisms affect the tempo and rate at which a person redefines and relates in alternative ways. The cyclical nature of these interactions is summarized in Figure 8-1, the interaction of identity, relating, and control in maintenance of mental health.

Challenges to older individuals and their families, specific concerns, and interventions have been discussed throughout this text. There is, however, scant evidence that "general mental health" can be directly promoted or strengthened in order to prevent severe mental disorders (Lamb & Zusman, 1981). Primary prevention of psychological distress in aging consists of reeducation of the public in regard to the aging process. Secondary prevention consists of identification and treatment of disease (Hendricks & Hendricks, 1977).

Martin (1970) argues that primary prevention is unattainable and that secondary prevention is enough. In reality, prevention of psychological distress in aging involves largely secondary measures aimed at control of precipitants rather than causative factors in mental illness. Nonetheless, even secondary efforts aimed at prevention of unnecessary deterioration of psychosocial competence are valid enough to warrant continuation. Prevention efforts directed at strengthening and maintaining the older individual's identity, relating, and control over environmental challenges and threats appear to be a logical approach.

PREVENTION AND MAINTENANCE THROUGH PUBLIC EDUCATION

Schaie (1981) identified three broad areas of special importance to wellness and maintenance of mental health in the aged and their families. These areas are (1) reeducation of the public sector, especially the media, relative to successful aging; (2) health education of the older individual relative to normal and atypical biopsychosocial changes in functional abilities; and (3) preretirement education including leisure counseling to facilitate the transition from the world of work to the world of enforced leisure.

The absence of meaningful vocational or leisure opportunities and resulting role constriction are amplified by the bigotry of ageism. These social realities diminish later-life satisfaction and depreciate possible contributions of the "terminally old."

Popular opinion encourages the elderly to "keep busy" in order to maintain wellness; however, there are few clear prescriptions for how and at what the older person is supposed to keep busy (Foner & Schwab, 1981). Even the non-scientific "use it or lose it" attitude is acceptable as long as there are meaningful options for discharging productive energy. Otherwise, the attitude itself becomes a source of stress and frustration for families and older members. Satisfying later-life adjustment is possible, but there are a number of barriers to overcome. Educational efforts must be marshaled on all fronts simultaneously. The attitudes of the public sector and the older person's beliefs about his or her own aging must be challenged and changed.

The public sector's experience with normal and atypical aging is limited by inexperience and circumscribed by stereotyping. Some of the stereotypes are more damaging than others but all do a disservice. McKenzie (1980, pp. 9–16) identifies several stereotypes that currently undermine the psychosocial competence of older persons. Three of the most damaging stereotypes that require reeducation are as follows:

1. Aging means homogeneity, reflected in the widespread belief that as people grow older they lose individuality and become more alike. In fact, older persons are less alike than groups of younger people. With advanced age, the personality increasingly differentiates so that diversity and individuality are more the rule than the exception (Maddox & Douglas, 1974).

2. Aging means senility. Whereas all persons are susceptible to cognitive and psychosocial impairments along the life span, aging does appear to increase the probability of cognitive difficulties, especially problems with memory. However, it has been repeatedly demonstrated that many cases of cognitive impairments are secondary to other problems such as depression, nutrition, and general physical health.

3. Aging brings rigidity, inflexibility, and contrariness. Some studies do suggest that older persons change attitudes and behaviors somewhat more

slowly than younger people, but the changes that must be accommodated are incredible at this stage of life. Moreover, in many cases, there are few opportunities for older persons to select the new over the traditional.

Inflexibility is implied in the popular belief that "you can't teach an old dog new tricks." Birren, Butler, Greenhouse, Sokoloff, and Yarrow (1963) conducted longitudinal research to determine changes in the developmental learning of aptitudes. They concluded that while there is some slowing in psychological and physiological reaction of time taken to process information, the ability or capacity to learn does not decrease in healthy older people.

Botwinick (1973) found that the patterns of adjustment and social behaviors of normal aged do not vary significantly from individuals in other age groups. Actually, given the stresses of aging, it is amazing that older people are not significantly more negative and hostile than other age groups. Other troublesome stereotypes include the belief that older people are sexless, more serene, more religious, less creative, and always lonely (McKenzie, 1980).

The term *ageism* was coined by Robert Butler (1969), a psychiatrist, to describe the prejudice surrounding aging. "Ageism reflects a deep-seated uneasiness on the part of the young and middle aged—a personal revulsion to and distaste for growing old, disease, disability and fear of powerlessness, 'uselessness' and death" (p. 245). Butler perceived ageism as a serious threat to wellness and successful adjustment in later life. He cautioned that as a force ageism is not readily amenable to redirection. Certainly, the media have done little to aid the redirection. Research, though limited, indicates that the elderly are portrayed on television in negative, stereotypical ways (Marshall & Wallenstein, 1973).

In a random sampling of all types of television programs, Harris and Feinberg (1978) found that there were few positive portrayals of effective old people, sexuality was absent, and poor health was a frequent theme. Ansello (1978) found that the elderly were depicted as unengaging and were used especially in commercials advocating the "tried and true" characteristics of a variety of products. Hess and Markson (1980) concluded that television and novels depict few positive features of old age to offset the dreary tedium of growing old in our society. Clearly, educational efforts must increase the public's understanding of aging. Awareness of the many positive aspects of aging must be heightened. The myths and stereotypes that themselves are incapacitating, self-fulfilling prophecies for older Americans must be dispelled and eliminiated.

Old age then should be publicly represented as one developmental phase within the human life span. Many of the secondary symptoms of pathological aging result from a variety of factors, including environment deficiencies, stresses, and social stereotyping, that can be eliminated through remediation of the public mind.

PREVENTION AND MAINTENANCE THROUGH HEALTH EDUCATION

Maintenance of mental health and wellness requires an older individual to define the physical self as it relates to the environment, including health care professionals, in a responsible manner. Schaie (1981) identifies health education as an important feature in wellness and maintenance of mental health. Many believe the old adage, "a healthy body makes for a healthy mind."

The directive to provide health education and information to older people is, however, a grossly underestimated task. In reality, health professionals and academicians have offered public service lecture series on common health problems. However, little exploration of older individuals' experiences, perceptions, and understandings has been accomplished. Doctor visits tend to be brief. Responsibility for education in direct health service provision falls to others.

Review of the task of educating an older person about his or her physical health and physical maintenance in light of multiple treatment and medication regimes and physical limitations, given multiple chronic illnesses, appears overwhelming. Yet additional educational tasks include outlining the warning signs of acute illnesses, side effects of medications, illness causation, progression of illness, and expected treatment outcomes. It is not surprising that medical systems have historically sidestepped the issue by becoming authoritarian and directive with older individuals: "Take one of these pills three times a day with meals. Come back in six months. Call me if you have any problems."

The challenge then is how to approach older people who are greatly in need of education about health issues and treatments, provide meaningful health information, and subsequently impact their quality of life. The most practical approach may be through open discussion with the older individual about his or her perceptions of symptoms, diagnosis, and treatment. The value of this approach is clear in the following case.

A 78-year-old widower living alone in the community called to request a home visit. He identified problems of Parkinson's disease and vaguely hinted of depression and loneliness. At his home, he was confined to a chair due to inertia problems, rigidity, and arthritis that allowed him to rise from a sitting position only with great physical effort and persistence. Despite these limitations, he lived alone with only a part-time homemaker three days a week.

During the home visit, he immediately launched into a discussion about how to obtain a tincture of strychnine. He was well aware that strychnine was a poison; however, he firmly believed that this tincture with a very small amount of strychnine could help his Parkinson's disease. When asked to elaborate, he described a lifelong interest in home remedies, herbs, teas, and natural vitamins. He described an early-life fascination with pharmacies and their products. He also described frustration with doctors and treatments that had unsuccessfully managed his chronic, progressive disease. He had single-handedly cared for his invalid wife during the early years of his Parkinson's disease. She had suffered a great deal of discomfort and pain the last years of her life as a result of an unsuccessful surgical repair of repeated hip fractures. Again, his frustration was directed at physicians who "botched the surgeries."

After ventilation of these concerns, he was then able to explain that he truly believed the strychnine from the nux vomica plant would work on his nervous system. He felt that it would stimulate better function and control of his legs, which of course were limiting his function. He had major difficulties accepting his chronic illness and the limitations of current treatments. He chose to fantasize about the past when a variety of pharmaceuticals and potions had controlled all the physical ailments in his youth.

At other times, patients may resist such extensive elaboration or be unable to articulate their concerns and past experiences so clearly. Creative attempts to understand their perceptions and misunderstandings may be necessary as in the following case.

An 82-year-old widow was admitted to the hospital for chronic, mild drug abuse of aspirin, over-the-counter pain medications, and nerve preparations. She insisted that she needed something for her "nerves" and was obsessed about lack of control of her nervousness. She was then asked to draw a picture of her nervous system. Her drawing consisted of many small, frayed, disconnected, swiggly lines that she felt represented her "nerves." She pointed out how a doctor had told her she had "sensitive nerve endings," which she included in the drawing. Surprisingly, there was no noticeable connection of her peripheral nervous system to her brain. Education about the central nervous system control over "nerves" and reinforcement of her ability to integrate her own "frazzled nerves" was then possible. She readily accepted new information about her health when it was related to her current perceptions and misunderstandings.

Practical experience outlines the process of educating older people about health concerns. The task begins with exploration of their current understanding of the symptoms, causes, and treatments; their past health education; and interest as well as their past experience with health care providers either directly or indirectly through experiences of the family. It is this complex array of perceptions and experiences that influences current approaches to health care. Misunderstandings may be common. Noncompliance with treatment regimes and medications may be rampant.

Another widely recognized dilemma of the health educator is that knowledgeable individuals display no change in their health behaviors. Clearly many individuals know that smoking causes cancer and lung disease; obesity is related to heart disease, hypertension, and diabetes; and salt is related to hypertension. However, these same knowledgeable people continue to smoke, overeat, and use salt. Knowledge is not always the variable that affects behavior.

For older individuals, the only solution lies in repeated educational efforts, appreciation of the idiosyncratic and unique health and illness perceptions of older individuals, and continued support through health maintenance clinics. Older people seem to want a clear understanding of the threat of their disease as well as information on how to cope with it. The challenge is getting this information to them in a useful, meaningful way.

ADJUSTMENTS IN LATER LIFE

Later-life adjustment to widowhood or retirement (see Chapter 5) is often characterized by discontinuities and constrictions in roles. These changes represent clear challenges to the identity, relating, and control of older individuals. Retirement is a common transition that must be carefully scripted in order to avoid unnecessary stress and ensure adaptation. Grandparenting opportunities can occur at various points along the life span, but most generally this role becomes significant in later life. Satisfaction, role enhancement, and new identity can occur in grandparenting, but is too often minimized by stereotyping. It is discussed in this section as an example of continuity of identity and expansion of relationship opportunities in later life.

Role Enhancement: Grandparenting

Individuals encounter grandparenting early in their own life cycle as grandchildren and again in later life as grandparents themselves. Consequently, the role of grandparenting spans the life cycle. Neugarten and Weinstein (1964) investigated the personal significance of grandparenthood and reported that five categories of psychosocial role meaning are apparent. The role and status is perceived as a source of biological renewal, as an opportunity to succeed in a different family role, and to achieve vicariously, as a teacher-resource role and as a remote role.

Clearly then, grandparenting represents an opportunity to expand later-life roles, and it is a major affective bridge between different life stages within a family life cycle. Family linkage is of crucial importance to the older individual (Adams, 1971; Sussman, 1976). Butler and Lewis (1976) conclude that a sense of relatedness is essential to maintenance of an identity as a significant human being. The grandparent role provides this sense. Kivnick (1982) systematically examined the grandparent role as it relates to later-life wellness and mental health. This research empirically demonstrates that older persons use the normative pathway of grandparenting to enhance their mental health. Kivnick (1982) reports the following results: "Clinical consideration of grandparenthood life histories suggested that throughout the life cycle generationally appropriate grandparenthood related experience contributes to the success with which an individual is able to resolve developmentally successive psychosocial conflicts" (p. 63). Successful grandparenting apparently contributes to psychosocial well-being throughout the life span, and it is an important developmental aspect of family mental health that is too often dismissed as folklore.

Current instability of the family structure revealed in the rates of divorce, remarriage, and blended families may undermine this important role expression for future grandparents. However, for the time being, the role of grandparenting is a valuable opportunity for the elderly to maintain continuity in relational patterns. The splitting of family units has prompted 21 states to enact laws protecting visitation rights of grandparents if in the best interest of the child (Wilson & DeShane, 1982). Nonetheless, confusion continues to surround the legal issues of grandparent rights. However, Wilson and DeShane (1982, p. 71) report the remarks of one grandparent who was denied access to her grandchildren. This reflection sums up the key issue of intergenerational continuity in the grandparenting role: ' "The judge can say anything he wants to. But I'll still be their grandmother. I'll be their grandmother until the day I die. Nothing can change that.' "

Role Constriction: Retirement

Role constriction as a result of the individual defining himself or herself as "retired" and of the work environment limiting relationships is a complex change. The legal mandatory retirement age was raised to age 70 in 1978, thereby increasing the individual's control over retirement by five years. However, the trend among Americans has been an earlier and earlier retirement age (Foner & Schwab, 1981). While current economics may change retirement patterns, most working Americans agree that "nobody should be forced to retire because of age, if he wants to continue working and is still able to do a good job and most Americans want to retire but they want the option of working part time instead of making a sharp change in role and status" (Louis Harris & Associates, 1981, pp. 8–10).

Clearly retirement is a life event that might be expected to cause problems in later-life adjustment. Work is important for psychological and physiological well-being (Liem & Liem, 1978). Riley and Waring (1976) note that serious role discontinuities often result from the abruptness of retirement.

There is an overall "lack of preparedness" for retirement especially among lower income, minority, and less-educated workers. Individuals least able to cope with ensuing financial and emotional hardships are also the least likely to be preparing for retirement (Louis Harris & Associates, 1981). For today's worker there are few role models from which to learn successful retiring. Lack of role continuity and lack of role clarity lead to significant role constriction for many. The loss of prestige and power, loss of established routines, and loss of social contacts greatly diminish the older person's identity and self-esteem, sense of "effectance," and sense of connection to the larger social mainstream.

Preretirement counseling and planning hopefully can lead to more positive adjustment in retirement transitions and prevent unnecessary role constrictions. Preretirement counseling helps the older worker anticipate the changes that can be expected upon retirement. Brower (1981) identifies a number of changes for which individuals should be prepared in *Hope: The Pre-Retirement Planning Guide,* including changes in life routine and responsibilities, changes in attitudes, and changes in relational patterns with one's retired or working spouse and other family members.

Preretirement planning generally focuses on education of the worker although some programs offer counseling along with educational services. For example, Action for Independent Maturity (AIM), a packaged preretirement program, consists of the following topics: (1) challenges of retirement, (2) health and safety, (3) housing, (4) legal affairs, (5) attitudes and role adjustment, (6) meaningful use of leisure time, and (7) sources of income and financial planning. (Information about AIM seminars can be obtained from Action for Independent Maturity, 1909 K Street, N.W., Washington, D.C. 20049. Information concerning *The Pre-Retirement Planning Guide* can be obtained from Hope Publishing and Training Center, Inc., 2040 N. 50th Avenue, Omaha, Nebraska 68104.)

Psychological distress may or may not be an automatic adjustment to retirement. Studies conducted with retired people reveal that the majority are satisfied (Foner & Schwab, 1981). Other research shows that 27 percent of older Americans are "living the promise of the golden years," 53 percent are finding life for the most part satisfactory, and 20 percent are casualties of poor health, economic strain, and loneliness (Weinstein, 1980).

In a current effort to "keep busy" and keep the older person active and consequently happy, "pseudowork" in the form of volunteerism is gaining popularity but not necessarily among the ranks of older retired workers. "Compensatory" leisure is another popular solution to anticipated adjustment difficulties associated with retirement. Supposedly it allows an individual to compensate for the lack of meaningfulness in work through leisure activity (Wilenski, 1960). Pseudowork and compensatory leisure do not significantly increase later-life adjustment because life satisfaction is much more complex than vocational or avocational matters. Leisure and recreational counseling are emerging approaches to increasing later-life adjustment beyond the simplicity of the keep-busy stereotype of retirement.

RECREATION AND LEISURE

Recreation and leisure activity are important to wellness and mental health throughout the life span. In addition, recreation and leisure provide some of the most creative ways for older individuals to structure relationships in the environment that support healthy redefinition of self and promote increased awareness of self. Middle-aged individuals who value their present leisure and recreation habits also project positive anticipation of a leisure life style during retirement (Balthaser & Farrell, 1981). Therefore, it is necessary to program meaningful leisure activities during midlife to ensure continuation of healthy leisure in later life. In this case the folk belief that "you don't stop playing because you grow old; you grow old because you stop playing" is shared by senior recreation specialists.

Nonetheless, large numbers of older people are not involved in meaningful recreation or their involvement is seriously limited. The perceived constraints on involvement are numerous but not insurmountable. Studies reveal that lack of physical ability, lack of leisure companions, lack of transportation, lack of money, fear of crime, lack of facilities, physical barriers, poor health, the weather, and fear of injury are the primary reasons senior citizens offer for lack of meaningful recreation (McGuire, 1981). Older individuals, especially impaired persons, as noted throughout this text are more susceptible to environmental influences. One leisure counseling program, Total Environment Approach (T.E.A.) was designed to eliminate limiting leisure factors by adapting physical, social, and psychological environments in which recreation occurs.

The physical setting was designed to accommodate sensory and motor loss; geographical proximity was considered along with transportation options; and activities based on stereotypes such as bingo were eliminated from the program. The perspective offered in the Total Environment Approach (McGuire, 1981) requires a change in the way that public programs and older persons perceive the leisure and recreational needs of later life.

The amount of enforced leisure in the lives of retired and older Americans necessitates much more active leisure, educational, and outreach counseling than currently available. Leisure counseling has been used for therapeutic and other purposes for older persons, including those with impairments (Loesch, 1981). Therefore, appropriate and effective leisure goals are available for any older person in any life circumstance. The traditional work ethic continues to pervade the thinking of many older people; enforced leisure can cause adjustment difficulties if not addressed along with other psychosocial competencies in mental health.

Physical well-being and general health are repeatedly found to be major influences in later-life satisfaction. Planned recreational activities can be utilized to maintain physical, mental, and social fitness and increase stress-resistiveness (Seleen, 1981). The goals of leisure education for the elderly are to identify those leisure activities that will be most satisfying and contribute to overall life satisfaction as well as develop leisure activities that will help an individual change (improve) in some specific way (Loesch, 1981). Leisure in this context is considered an important component of an older person's total wellness and mental health. There are approaches to leisure education that emphasize the similarities between work and leisure and approaches that emphasize the differences. However, approaches that emphasize the respective independencies of work and leisure appear to be the most relevant for counseling this generation of older persons (Allen, 1980) and assuring satisfaction with recreation and leisure activities.

SUMMARY

Mental health is more than the absence of mental illness. Support and maintenance of good mental health as well as prevention of mental illness must proceed. Stereotypes and popular attitudes that challenge an older person's definition of self, relating, and control must be countered with public education.

Americans aged 65 and older are not a homogeneous, undiversified group. Their circumstances vary with income, age, race, ethnicity, sex, personality, and the meaning assigned to varied life-span experiences. Too many elderly accept the marginal adjustment growing from the narrow, negative definition of aging behavior. Although the prevalence of psychological distress is reportedly near epidemic proportions, the elderly remain by and large a psychiatrically unobserved minority. The best hope for healthy aging resides in increased understanding of the impact of the family milieu as well as in increased education of the public sector and aging individuals. Such education would introduce the notion of accepting imperfections and change throughout the life-span development. Positive relationships with the current older population, personality integration, and sensitivity to their need for balance and control will surely affect the mental health of future generations of older people in healthy ways.

REFERENCES

Adams, D.L. Correlates of satisfaction among the elderly. *Gerontologist,* 1971, *11,* 64-68.

Allen, L.R. Leisure and its relationship to work and career guidance. *Vocational Guidance Quarterly,* 1980, *28* (3), 257-262.

Ansello, E.F. *Broadcast images: The older woman in television* (Part 1). Paper presented at the annual meeting of the Gerontological Society, Dallas, 1978.

Balthaser, B.A., & Farrell, P. Program recreation services for positive aging. *Parks & Recreation,* December 1981, pp. 35-36.

Birren, J.E., Butler, R.N., Greenhouse, S.W., Sokoloff, L., & Yarrow, M. (Eds.), *Human aging: A biological and behavioral study* (National Institutes of Health, PHS Publication no. 986). Washington, D.C.: U.S. Government Printing Office, 1963.

Botwinick, J. *Aging and behaviors.* New York: Springer Publishing, 1973.

Brower, H.C. *Hope: The preretirement planning guide.* Omaha: Hope Publishing and Training Center, 1981.

Butler, R.N. Ageism: Another form of bigotry. *Gerontologist,* 1969, *14,* 243-249.

Butler, R.N., & Lewis, M. *Aging and mental health.* St. Louis: C.V. Mosby, 1976.

Erikson, E.H. Identity and the life cycle. *Psychological issues,* 1959, *1* (1) (monograph). New York: International Universities Press, 1959.

Foner, A., & Schwab, K. *Aging and retirement.* Monterey, Calif.: Brooks/Cole, 1981.

Harris, A.J., & Feinberg, J. Television and aging: Is what you see what you get? *Gerontologist,* 1978, *18,* 422-426.

Harris L., & Associates. *Aging in the eighties: America in transition* (Survey highlights and fact sheets). Washington D.C.: The National Council on Aging, 1981.

Hendricks, J., & Hendricks, C.D. *Aging in mass society: Myths and realities.* Cambridge: Winthrop, 1977.

Hess, B.B., & Markson, E.W. *Aging and old age: An introduction to social gerontology.* New York: Macmillan Publishing, 1980.

Kivnick, H.Q. Grandparenthood: An overview of meaning and mental health. *Gerontologist,* 1982, *22,* 59-66.

Lamb, H.R., & Zusman, J. A new look at primary prevention. *Hospital and Community Psychiatry,* 1981, *32* (12), 843-848.

Liem, R., & Liem, J. Social class and mental illness reconsidered: The role of economic stress and social support. *Journal of Health and Social Behaviors,* 1978, *19,* 139-156.

Loesch, L.C. Leisure counseling for disabled older persons. *Journal of Rehabilitation,* October/November/December 1981, pp. 58-63.

Maddox, G., & Douglas, E. Aging and individual differences. *Journal of Gerontology,* 1974, *29,* 555-563.

Marshall, C., & Wallenstein, E. Beyond Marcus Welby, Cable TV for the health of the elderly. *Geriatrics,* 1973, *28,* 182-186.

Martin, L.E. *Mental health/Mental illness: Revolution in progress.* San Francisco: McGraw-Hill, 1970.

McGuire, F.A. Freedom to choose: The total environment approach. *Parks & Recreation,* December 1981, pp. 51-55.

McKenzie, S.C. *Aging and old age.* Glenview, Ill. Scott, Foresman and Company, 1980.

Neugarten, B.L., & Weinstein, K. The changing American grandparent. *Journal of Marriage and the Family,* 1964, *26,* 199–204.

Riley, M.W., & Waring, J. Age and aging. In R.K. Merton & R. Nisbet (Eds.), *Contemporary Social Problems* (4th ed.). New York: Harcourt Brace Jovanovich, 1976.

Schaie, K.W. Psychological changes from midlife to early old age: Implications for the maintenance of mental health. *American Journal of Orthopsychiatry,* 1981, *51,* 199–218.

Seleen, D.R. Senior swim: A healthful leisure program. *Parks & Recreation,* December 1981, pp. 57–60.

Sussman, M.B. The family life of old people. In R.H. Binstock & E. Shanas (Eds.), *Handbook of aging and the social sciences.* New York: Van Nostrand Reinhold, 1976.

Verwoerdt, A. *Clinical geropsychiatry.* Baltimore: Waverly Press, 1981.

Weinberg, J. Of slings and arrows and outrageous fortune. *The American Journal of Psychoanalysis,* 1979, *39,* 195–210.

Weinstein, G.W. You and retirement: Studies of older Americans. *The Elks Magazine,* September 1980, p. 35.

Wilenski, H.L. Work, careers and social integration. *International Social Science Journal,* 1960, *12,* 543–560.

Wilson, K.B., & DeShane, M.R. The legal rights of grandparents: A preliminary discussion. *Gerontologist,* 1982, *22,* 67–71.

Index

221

About the Authors

DONNA R. EYDE, Ph.D., earned a B.A. degree in anthropology and an M.Ed. degree from the University of Nebraska. In 1977, she was awarded a Ph.D. in special education and psychology from the University of Missouri at Columbia. She currently is an associate professor of educational therapy in the department of psychiatry at the University of Nebraska Medical Center. Dr. Eyde has considerable experience in a wide-range of special education fields, including working with behaviorally disordered children and providing services and counseling for the elderly and their families. As part of her work with the elderly, she established the Alzheimer's Disease Family Support Group of Omaha and served as coordinator of a workshop in Omaha on aging, anger, and the family.

JAY A. RICH, M.D., is a community psychiatrist in private practice in Omaha. He earned a B.S. degree from North Dakota State University and an M.D. in 1976 from the University of North Dakota. Much of his work has focused on mental health issues as they affect the family and community. He currently is pursuing a music degree connected with his research in music therapy.